Hysterectomy?
The *Best* or *Worst* Thing
That Ever Happened to Me?

Elizabeth Plourde, C.L.S., M.A.

New Voice Publications

PUBLISHER'S NOTE:

Some names used to identify an individual in the text of this book are pseudonyms only.

AN IMPORTANT CAUTION TO OUR READERS:

This book is not a medical manual and cannot take the place of personalized medical advice and treatment from a qualified physician. The reader should regularly consult a physician in matters relating to his or her health, particularly with respect to any symptoms that may require diagnosis or treatment. Although certain medical procedures and medical professionals are mentioned in this book, no endorsement, warranty or guarantee by the author is intended. Every attempt has been made to ensure that the information contained in this book is current, however, due to the fact that research is ongoing, some of the material may be invalidated by new findings. The author and publisher cannot guarantee that the information and advice in this book are safe and proper for every reader. For that reason, this book is sold without warranties or guarantees of any kind, expressed or implied, and the author and publisher disclaim any liability, loss or damage caused by the contents. If you do not wish to be bound by these cautions and conditions, you may return your copy to the publisher for a full refund.

Plourde, Elizabeth
Hysterectomy? The best or worst thing that ever happened to me? /
Elizebeth Plourde

ISBN 0-9661735-4-6
LCCN 2002117825

Cover design: Christy Salinas

Published by
New Voice Publications
P.O. Box 14133
Irvine, CA 92623-4133
www.newvoice.net
publisher@newvoice.net

This book is dedicated to:

All the millions of women around the world who have undergone removal of their uterus or ovaries. May your collective and varied experiences contribute toward a greater understanding of the female body and its wonderfully complex uniqueness, spurring improved health care for all the generations to come.

Acknowledgments

My deepest gratitude goes to all the women throughout the years who, by opening their hearts and sharing their wide range of experiences, made this book possible. Their words will not only help others to make informed choices, they will help to create an awareness of the complexity and individuality of our bodies, which hopefully will lead researchers to broaden their studies on women's health.

It was very hard to settle on the final story count, as each women's account is unique and all deserve to be heard. For the many who have written and are not on these pages, your words have not gone unheard. Even though time and resources demanded that I not include everyone, all your experiences have helped to guide me toward my next areas of research.

A special thank you to Drs. William H. Parker, Charles Coddington III, Herbert A. Goldfarb, and Elizabeth Lee Vliet for supporting this work with their very thoughtful contributions. I additionally thank Drs. Christiane Northrup, Jennifer R. Berman, and Laura A. Berman for their wonderful words of endorsement. Women's health care is changing and these foresighted doctors are helping to shape the face of the new medical model that is emerging—a model that recognizes our individual uniqueness, that one size (one procedure) does not fit all.

I also extend my gratitude to the many women who are working diligently towards improving the state of women's health care and providing forums for education, so women can be truly informed as they make crucial decisions regarding their health.

—Elizabeth Plourde - 2003

TABLE OF CONTENTS

Introduction

This book is dedicated to bringing an awareness to the realization that reproductive organ removal is a gamble. It contains a collection of letters I have received from hysterectomized women over the 16 years that I have been researching, writing, and lecturing about these surgeries, and hormone replacement therapy. As I read these letters, I felt the world needed to hear the heartfelt words women from around the world use when they are describing how their lives have changed since their surgery.

One hundred years of medical studies clearly show that approximately 1/3 of women are adversely affected in some way by their hysterectomy. The 2/3s who are not affected, and feel their hysterectomy "was the best thing that ever happened to them" are why doctors have not been able to understand the 1/3 who DO develop symptoms, and why they keep recommending and performing over 600,000 hysterectomies every year in the United States alone. Women cannot know beforehand, however, if they will be one of the lucky ones whose problems are corrected, without developing side effects, or be one of the ones whose lives are devastated.

Every year millions of women throughout the world, who are not facing life-threatening conditions such as cancer or childbirth complications, are told they need a hysterectomy. In many instances they are advised that it is their only avenue of relief. Often they are not informed about the many seemingly unrelated consequences that can arise as a result of losing their uterus and/or ovaries. I cannot begin to estimate the number of women who have called or written to me about the new problems that have arisen from their surgery stating: "My doctor never told me," or "I was assured there would be no change in my sexual response, and now I feel nothing." Even if women try researching prior to their decision, it is very difficult to read dry medical statistics of potential outcomes and feel that any of these outcomes could happen to them. While reading that 1/3 to 1/2 of women experience depression afterwards, it is easy to think, "I won't be one of them." Since the surgery cannot be undone, women deserve to know about all the possible outcomes, as well as have the risks of cancer put into the proper perspective, so they can make truly informed decisions. Having hysterectomized women tell how their lives have been changed will help those needing to decide whether having surgery is the right path for them and their particular circumstances, before undergoing such a body and life altering procedure.

This book will also help the millions of women around the world, including the 30 million in the United States, who have already undergone a hysterectomy, and may be experiencing difficulties from either structural changes or symptoms of hormone deprivation. Many symptoms occur from the ovaries being removed, or compromised as a result of the uterus being removed. Medical studies clearly indicate that 20% of the time the ovaries shut down when the uterus is removed. When one ovary is removed, the remaining ovary shuts down 33% of the time. Many of these women were not informed of this potential outcome. I have received many letters thanking me for my first book: *Your Guide to Hysterectomy, Ovary Removal, & Hormone Replacement*. Women state: "I now know that I am not alone." "I now know that I am not crazy." "I now know there is help available." "I now know there is hope." These women provide us with such a consistent constellation of symptoms, they can no longer be ignored. There are biochemical explanations for all of the symptoms these women exhibit, with 1,000s of medical studies supporting the fact that these new conditions CAN arise. Sadly, however, many of these women are offered only a referral to a psychiatrist when their symptoms are not understood.

As I started compiling the stories, I realized that the women who said it was the "best thing that ever happened to them" were primarily women who had only their uterus removed. Their immediate problems were resolved. There are also many fortunate women who never develop problems later. It became clear that the hysterectomized women who are most adversely affected are those who also had either one or both of their ovaries removed, or had them compromised by the surgery, creating instant menopause. These women can suffer debilitating damage and many are not able to find the help they need to fully recover. They have spent years behind closed doors, so debilitated that they are unable to get out of the house. Their stories reveal the great disruption ovary removal, or impairment of ovarian function, has on the rest of body, a disruption that has not been recognized or honored up to this point. Loss of ovarian function, however, is the major change that many of these women have in common. Oophorectomized (ovaries removed) women are the ones who suffer year in and year out, attempting to regain the health they had prior to surgery. As a result, this is a major division in the book. Part One includes women who have had only a hysterectomy. Part Two is women who have had one ovary removed. Part Three is women who have had both ovaries removed. Part Four is experiences provided by family members. Part Five represents women who had a tubal ligation prior to a hysterectomy. I included this section because I heard from so many women who recognized their hormonal imbalance symptoms began shortly after their tubal ligation. Part 6 is women I heard from for whom hysterectomy was recommended, but they were able to obtain resolution of their symptoms without having to resort to surgery.

A greater recognition that nonsurgical solutions are possible is of critical importance. Any surgery, even though many have great outcomes, can lead to new problems that can compromise women's health more than the conditions they were trying to correct. Even the women who feel their uterus removal was the

best thing that ever happened to them are still subject to the
future potential of a cystocele (bladder herniating or falling and
pressing against front wall of vagina), rectocele (rectum pushing
against back wall of vagina), or vaginal vault prolapse (vagina
turning inside out and falling out the vaginal opening), all of
which can be outcomes of surgical invasion of the organs and
their supporting structures. They can also develop adhesions,
so painful that they require additional surgeries in an attempt to
alleviate the pain, only to develop more adhesions due to the
new surgery. Other new conditions can even include bowel
incontinence, which leads to these women being placed on 100%
disability for the rest of their lives.

At this beginning of the 21st century, there needs to be a
change in how we view the body and how western medicine is
practiced. Up to now, women's reproductive organs have
been viewed as parts that were easily expendable if they were not
functioning quite right. The surgical outcome, however, has left
millions of women attempting to function with valuable pieces
missing—pieces that are needed to attain and maintain vibrant
health. There are no pieces put into our bodies that are not
necessary. The standard medical practice of removing perfectly
healthy functioning ovaries needs to be re-examined in the
light of today's biochemical evidence, as well as the testimonials
from women around the world.

Loss of the valuable hormones and chemicals secreted by
the ovaries results in a greater risk of heart disease (women's #1
killer) and osteoporosis, which combined kill 550,000 women
every year. Since the ovarian hormones interact with every other
system in the body, hysterectomized women are also subjected to
metabolic changes over which they have no control, resulting in
a gain or loss of weight. They experience problems with unclear
thinking and memory loss. The hormonal imbalance can also
lead to difficult to treat problems such as fibromyalgia and
osteoarthritis. Women are treated for these problems without

the recognition that the surgical disruption of their finely tuned hormonal system led to these disease states.

A man's testicles create sperm and therefore, like ovaries, regenerate life on the planet. Does that mean men should have their testicles removed when they are through having all the children they want—just because there is a risk of testicular cancer? No! The medical community knows that men's bodies do not function the same if a man's testicles are removed, particularly in the sexual arena. So why does this same medical community consider that women's bodies will function the same when their ovaries are removed? The vast majority of the ovary removals in the United States are performed only out of the fear of cancer, not because a woman actually has ovarian cancer, which accounts for 26,000 new cases each year. In the United States, over 450,000 women lose their ovaries every year even though studies show that for approximately 1/3 of these women their ability to feel sexual is vastly hampered, if not completely obliterated.

Studies and research do not, for the most part, include the information as to whether a woman has had a hysterectomy or ovary removal when they have been diagnosed with any of the conditions that can occur due to hormonal disruption. All future research needs to include this data in order to get a clearer picture of the long-term consequences involved in disrupting the bodies natural hormonal ecosystem and the subsequent impact on women's health. However, the body is so complex and interrelated it will still be hard to determine how much of a role these surgeries play as there are myriad responses to the surgery depending on the reasons for the surgery, differences in surgical technique, and whether ovary function was disrupted.

In *Your Guide to Hysterectomy, Ovary Removal, & Hormone Replacement: What All Women Need to Know*, I outlined the biochemical reasons for the onset of heart disease, strokes, depression, fibromyalgia, osteoporosis, inability for the body to heal from accidents, bladder and bowel problems, and sexual dysfunction. The body is an intricate, highly complex machine. Changes in one area create changes in every other area throughout the body. This is precisely what happens with women who lose their ovarian hormones. The ovarian 17beta-estradiol performs many functions to assure that the arteries surrounding our hearts are not filled with plaque. It is also our body's built-in anti-depressant, performing the exact same job as most of the antidepressants that are on the market—that of increasing our body's level of serotonin, our "feel good" chemical. Its interaction with insulin assures that we maintain normal body weight and are not thrown into a diabetic condition. Our collagen and connective tissues are highly dependent upon estrogen. When we lose this precious chemical at menopause, we start to age and develop wrinkles and osteoarthritis. Estrogen is also essential for the health of the cells surrounding the bladder and vagina. Without it, vaginas can atrophy and bladder incontinence can become a problem.

The other ovarian hormones are also essential for our continued health. Testosterone is not just our sex drive hormone. It is essential in building and maintaining muscles, keeping them strong and toned. These strong muscles in turn play a role in protecting our joints. Our entire skeletal health is dependent on strong healthy muscles. Without strong muscles, our joints are stressed, resulting in more wear and tear, and there is difficulty in maintaining the proper alignment of our spinal column. Bone health is dependent on all three ovarian hormones: estradiol, progesterone, and testosterone.

When the health of surgically altered women starts to fail, their relationships fail, as husbands and mates get tired of the wife being constantly sick, in pain, and in multiple doctors' offices seeking relief from their symptoms. Their relationships with their children suffer, as they lose the ability to be patient with them, or physically cannot take care of them any more. In many ways their personalities change so much, they are no longer emotionally able to be there for either their children or their husbands.

With the preliminary results of the Women's Health Initiative (WHI) being published in July of 2002 proving that replacement of ovarian hormones is not as easy as was originally thought, it is even more imperative to hear the words of the women on these pages who have suffered loss of their ovaries. Women can no longer be assured that all they have to do is take an estrogen pill every day to replace what is either removed or compromised by surgery.

Women, become informed prior to making any health care decisions, especially major surgery. Many women have told me over the years that they did not know much about their body before surgery, but as they sought to find answers for their new medical problems, they now know more than they ever wanted to know about their body.

The experiences in this book are not just isolated cases, they all have the potential of occurring many times every day as these surgeries continue to be performed by the 100s of thousands for non-life-threatening reasons. These letters are offered in the hopes that removal of perfectly healthy ovaries will become an historical concept, and that due to the risk of ovarian dysfunction arising from the surgery, hysterectomies will be performed only in life threatening circumstances. It is also my hope that renewed efforts will go into women's research. When we decide that removing organs is no longer an option, new techniques and healing methods will provide solutions for the myriad problems that lead women to considering surgery in the first place—solutions that preserve the integrity of the reproductive organs—providing ALL women with the opportunity for life-long vibrant health.

—Elizabeth Plourde - 2003

Hysterectomy?

The *Best* or *Worst* Thing

That Ever Happened to Me?

What Doctors are Saying

Charles Coddington III, M.D.

This book raises very important and interesting points regarding what I believe are crucial parts to our current quality health care for women. The issue centers upon basic doctor and patient relationships and communication as well as clinical skill of the individual physician. As a teacher and mentor for numerous residents and students, one of the most important things that can be taught is the adage "know what you know and know what you don't know". The corollary to this is to refer or consult for assistance to gain expertise at the operating table when one is progressing to surgery and limits of capability may be tested. The other aspect is that of communicating to the patient what the disease process is and helping her come to a decision about care and procedures. This is extremely important. I have tried to use many different ways to engage patients in this process, having more success with some than others. It has been hard to convince them that they need to be a part of the decision because, after all, there are no guarantees nor is there any way to replace what is surgically removed. In some cases, trainees and other health care team members are part of this process by going over with the patient a second time what I have already covered in the counseling. My logic is not to burden the patient, but to have her hear it from another source—another human being, thus raising possible questions about the procedure or process. I do believe there are very few physicians practicing that would willfully do something wrong. I cannot validate this statement and neither can any of you, but the basic motivating force of each physician is one of service and caring, which is instilled in this group. As more and more pressure has been brought on the medical system and autonomous practice lessened, the students have chosen the medical profession from their inner drive and desire to contribute, rather than prestige or financial security. In fact, many of them will have to make many sacrifices and attain significant debts for the goal of becoming a physician.

So where am I going with these words introduction for this provocative text? I think this is a good mirror and reality check for us as practicing physicians and for patients as well. This publication is a recounting of individual experiences, which is worth reading and comprehending. Patients and professionals alike can learn from these examples of what went right or wrong. There are problems that will occur regardless of how excellent counselors we are or how skilled we are. We must communicate this to the patient. Every effort must be given to have the patient understand her options, and we, as professionals, must be accepting enough to embrace that choice, even if it does not involve surgery (as was the case for a number of women in the latter chapters). I feel many times I will talk to individuals and decide not to perform surgery more than I will convince them to have it. Although that seems to counter what one would think, it is true. I do clearly feel the more the patient understands and the more she hears, the less anxiety she has if surgery is decided upon. Clearly options of appropriate medical therapy need be tried, but not without follow-up or adjustments in care. An example was the use of Lupron to either increase the blood count (hematocrit) or to decrease the size of the uterine fibroids. This therapy does stop uterine bleeding, however it does have significant side effects. Many times patients have signs and symptoms of menopause. These can be treated by low dose estrogen replacement without compromising the effectiveness of the initial medicine. Physicians and patients need to communicate (which includes listening) when side effects begin to happen, particularly those less frequent symptoms that may be significant on the patient's quality of life.

I feel there are several steps that are imperative for the patient to explore when embarking on surgery or any other medical therapy. First, educate yourself about the procedure and the various ways in which one can be treated. One may ask, "how do I know or tell what's up"? One can go to web sites, such as that for the American College of Obstetricians and Gynecologists or to the site of subspecialty groups such as the American Society of Reproductive Medicine. This may require time or computer expertise, but I think that they are worth it. Secondly, one might obtain a second opinion. These do require time, but should not be costly. It is important to tell your doctor that you want another review and enlist her/his help. This fact is important because the doctor giving the second opinion will benefit from the records from the initial physician. If need be, have specific questions written when you go to the second opinion and write yourself notes to compare the two therapies. I feel, without a doubt, that it is worth the cost, even if you need to pay for it. Do not use the Internet for second opinions. There is no way to validate the credentials of the individual on the other end. Regardless of how well meaning someone is, it is always important to address the patient face to face if possible and examine the patient if that is what is needed. This can not be done, obviously, over the Internet. Managed care plans and Medicare will pay if there is a conflict between the two physicians, so that is important to note. Investigate for yourself whether your private insurance plan or Medicare will pay for the second opinion. Laws in approximately 42 states and the District of Columbia give the patients the right to an independent review in appealing a treatment decision by their HMO or managed care plan. As you can see, it is very important for the patient to become involved. Using the second opinion, it provides another perspective from which to hear the information. You can then formulate questions to ask the initial physician. The use of second opinions has become more frequent in my practice and is less threatening now than it might have been years ago. I'm sure there are some physicians who may be upset regarding the request for a second opinion, but if you feel it is worthwhile so be it. Another option would be to talk to other individuals and see what their experience has been; much like those contained in this publication. *It may not be your experience, but it is one place to gain information.* One has to weigh the opinions of other individuals, but you can find support groups to be of assistance as well. Thirdly, and most importantly, choose a physician you trust. One may have to rely on instinct, but this can be positive for you. Have they communicated well with you? Asked what you expect both preoperatively and postoperatively? This will be important to your well-being and allow planning for assistance postoperatively, if needed. Have an understanding of what to do if there is a question or problem. I feel that if a patient has a question or issue, it needs to be helped or resolved, at least as best we can. It may require you to write lists or notes—I would recommend you do so. Utilize some method that will remind you what needs to be done. Information on individual physicians can be gained by several local state medical societies, as far as their practice. I think the most important issue will be how the physician has treated others.

In summary, I think that there are many things that we can gain from this publication. They may center on physician and patient communication and relationships, as well as gaining a clear understanding of what the therapeutic process will be. I congratulate Elizabeth and her contributors in calling to our attention such important issues as these so that the quality of care rendered to the individual will be superb.

—Charles Coddington III, M.D.
　　Professor of Ob-Gyn University of Colorado Health Science Center
　　Director of OB-Gyn Denver Health Medical Center

Herbert A. Goldfarb, M.D.

This book is a powerful indictment of the potential side effects of hysterectomy. The old bromide that, "You've had your family and your uterus is only a source of problems" is obviously a misguided vestige of a time when physicians decided to treat hysteria by performing hysterectomy (the Freudian concept that all women's problems could be traced to sexuality gone astray).

Today we appreciate the devastation that unnecessary surgery has wrought. It behooves the modern mature woman to understand the problems they face, as well as and the modern medical alternatives to hysterectomy.

Almost all women over 35 years of age will experience irregular bleeding during their reproductive lives. This bleeding is called dysfunctional bleeding (after the Greek abnormal function). If they happen to have fibroids then many physicians will recommend hysterectomy to solve the problem. Many new alternative treatments to hysterectomy have been developed over the last fifteen years. Firstly, the physician should diagnose the cause of the bleeding by performing a hysteroscopy (looking inside the uterus). Small myomas can be removed at the same time. Other treatments for persistent bleeding includes various types of ablation (destroying the lining of the uterus to stop heavy bleeding). Uterine artery embolization, myolysis, uterine artery coagulation and varying types of myomectomy (removing only the fibroid tumor) can help save your uterus. For further information consult Ms. Plourde's first book *Your Guide to Hysterectomy, Ovary Removal, & Hormone Replacement:* or my book, *The No Hysterectomy Option.*

Medicine is like a huge ship. Even though it is changing direction and is beginning to turn around, we must remember that ships move very slowly and they cannot be turned on a dime. During this time of transition, women can advance their own cause best by heeding this paraphrase of a well known retailer, "Our best patient is an informed one."

—Herbert A. Goldfarb, M.D.
Director of Endoscopic Surgery, NYU Downtown Hospital
Author of *The No Hysterectomy Option*
hgoldfarb@viconet.com

William H. Parker, M.D.

Hysterectomy, the surgical removal of the uterus, is surrounded by controversy – and, for good reason. Every year, more than 600,000 American women have a hysterectomy, and almost 500,000 have their ovaries removed surgically. Moreover, the number of women who have a hysterectomy is expected to rise as the baby boom generation enters the ages when hysterectomy is most commonly performed. Already, by the age of 60, one out of every three women in the U.S. has had a hysterectomy. For individual women, and health care in general, hysterectomy is a vast and important issue.

Disturbingly, studies show that a lot of hysterectomies are unnecessary. For example, French doctors almost never perform a hysterectomy for fibroids, the most common reason given for the hysterectomies performed in the U.S. Also, women in the southern part of the U.S. are 78% more likely to have a hysterectomy than women who live in the Northeast. These differences suggest that factors other than good medical care are involved in a doctor's recommendation for a hysterectomy.

Yet, some women with intractable symptoms that affect their lives, may benefit from hysterectomy. One study found that most women who had a hysterectomy performed for moderate or severe symptoms were "very satisfied" with the results of surgery. It appears that if you are suffering from severe pain or bleeding, hysterectomy can sometimes offer improvement in the quality of your life. But how is a woman to know if the hysterectomy a doctor suggests is truly warranted? If you wish to keep your ovaries, are the risks of developing ovarian cancer overstated? Will you see any psychological or sexual differences after hysterectomy? Where do these issues leave the skeptical woman who is truly suffering and for whom a hysterectomy might provide a reasonable option? Are there other options for relief short of hysterectomy and major surgery?

Without a doubt, there are now many alternatives, both non-surgical and surgical, that can help many women avoid hysterectomy. Unfortunately, many gynecologists still do not offer these alternatives to women. Endometrial ablation, a simple outpatient procedure, is a very effective treatment for some women who are bleeding heavily. Myomectomy allows removal of just fibroids, with preservation of the uterus. Uterine fibroid embolization, a non-surgical procedure, is another effective treatment for many women with fibroids. Removal of an ovarian cyst, often using outpatient laparoscopic surgery, can be safely performed, instead of the more commonly performed procedure, removal of both ovaries and complete hysterectomy. Many other examples of under utilized alternatives exist.

This book contains stories from many women who have had hysterectomies, and others who also had their ovaries removed. The stories have been compiled and edited by Elizabeth Plourde, who, after the publication of her book, *Your Guide to Hysterectomy, Ovary Removal, & Hormone Replacement* received hundreds of letters and e-mails from women wanting to relate personal stories about their own experiences with surgery and the aftermath. Some women have found their surgery and recovery relatively easy, and have found relief from the pain or bleeding that controlled their lives and limited their activity. For these women, surgery was a good solution and the start of a new life.

—William Parker, M.D.
Author of *A Gynecologist's Second Opinion*
Clinical Professor, Department of Ob-Gyn UCLA School of Medicine
Vice-Chair, Department of Ob-Gyn Saint John's Medical Center

Elizabeth Lee Vliet, M.D.

Hysterectomy? The Best or Worst Thing that Ever Happened to Me? is an eloquent compilation of women's voices and women's stories about this deeply personal experience in a woman's life. I commend Elizabeth Plourde for her journey with other women to explore the ramifications—positive and negative—of this common surgery. It isn't a simple subject. Ms. Plourde's book delves into the complexities and nuances of how women can be affected at every level—physical, emotional, and spiritual—with the surgical removal of uterus and/or ovaries. As a *nonsurgeon* physician specializing in women's health for the last twenty years, and focusing my work on the incredible complexities of the multitudinous ways that our ovarian hormones are linked to the function of every cell and tissue of our bodies, I have personally treated several thousand women who have needed to find ways to restore optimal hormone health following pelvic surgeries such as hysterectomies. I spend hours researching the latest scientific research giving us new understandings about how our marvellous ovarian hormones oversee so many different functions of our bodies and brain-mind. I write books on the subject, I write medical papers on the subject, and I have taught seminars for health professionals and consumers around the country on these overlooked hormone connections in women's health and how crucial it is for those of us in medicine to take these issues seriously.

Yet, I write this not just as a physician and scientist. I write this as a woman who has been there, a woman who has had this surgery herself. I know what it is like to go through the tumultuous feelings of grief and loss, even when accepting the medical reasons for having the surgery. I know what it is like to experience surgical complications, and have to go back into the hospital yet again. Doctors often jokingly say that they do not like performing surgery on other doctors because whatever can go wrong usually does! Another "learning experience." Then too, I know what it is like to struggle to find hormone balance again. It isn't a simple matter. There is much to consider for women who are faced with whether or not to have a hysterectomy. No matter how needed the procedure, it IS a life-changing event—positive, negative, and all points in-between these opposites. Ms. Plourde's vignettes of women who have had hysterectomies allow you to peek inside their lives to see the many ways this is true at all levels of our being.

Today, there are many options to explore that may help you avoid having the surgery and women deserve better answers and discussion of such options than they have typically received in our fragmented, time-pressured health care system today. I describe many of these non-surgical options in my own books and seminars, and many resources are available to help women read more on these options. But what about the women who really have reached the end of available non-surgical options? What then? We *must* do a better job as health professionals to educate women about ways to avoid the horrible outcomes and painful experiences women describe in the pages ahead.

Today, many hysterectomies are now performed only when medical options have failed and there are very clear indications that it is needed, such as severe endometriosis, excessive bleeding, extremely painful periods, severe fibroids that cause abdominal distension and pain with intercourse, and uterine or ovarian cancer. However, there are still many women for whom hysterectomy is recommended as the only option, or the only one that will solve their problem. These women are not informed about the many new alternatives that have come to the forefront, leaving them to feel they have no choice except surgery. I feel strongly that women should be given information about the many non-surgical medication options today that can help alleviate such problems and in many cases prevent the need for surgery. I am shocked in my consultations, as one example, I often encounter women who have not been offered the simple option of trying different birth control pills to control pain, bleeding, endometriosis, and fibroids.

As far as hysterectomy's outcomes, conflicting results still abound in the medical literature. Some studies show hysterectomy can lead to depression, diminished self esteem, difficulty with sexual function, loss of bladder control, and a host of other problems. What isn't explained is that many of these problems result from poor hormone management AFTER surgery, rather than the surgery itself. More recent studies, when improved surgical techniques have been more widely used, show the opposite: depression (as a mood state, not the illness), is about half the incidence found prior to surgery, with women showing improved psychological and physical well being—including sexual enjoyment—after hysterectomy. We certainly see many patients who have low hormone levels and don't feel "back to normal" following a hysterectomy, but often these women are grateful the surgery took care of the bleeding or pain.

Why the discrepancy among the studies? Let's look at some crucial often overlooked facts.

1. Surgeons rarely measure hormone levels before surgery, when women feel well, to have a baseline for comparison later to determine whether the ovaries still produce the optimal hormone levels that are normal for her. Doctors just assume the ovaries continue to work fine after a surgery that removes only the uterus. In many women, they don't. Current studies have found that 30-60% of women have menopausal levels of estradiol and testosterone as early as two to three years following removal of the uterus. Insidious decline in ovarian hormone production wreaks havoc throughout our bodies, in every organ system, including the brain.

Most of these studies came from England, Germany, Italy, and other European countries. In the United States, this issue has not been taken as seriously. It is not clear to me why doctors here don't think follow-up checks of ovarian hormone levels are necessary. Dr. John Studd, an internationally known menopause researcher from London, is a strong advocate for follow-up tests of women's hormone levels after hysterectomy that leaves the ovaries. Dr. Studd says the majority of gynecologists and primary care physicians miss the diagnosis of premature hormonal decline after removal of only the uterus. He attributes the oversight in part to two factors: the loss of menstruation as a marker of the phases of the ovarian hormone cycle, and to doctors' *assumptions* that "vague" symptoms such as insomnia, anxiety, low libido, and depressed mood occur because of psychological reactions to losing the uterus, to feelings of lost femininity, or fear of aging. This focus on assumed psychological issues completely overlooks the physical hormone effects on brain chemistry. There is confirmation of this endocrine connection in such symptoms: FSH is elevated to menopausal levels in about 30% of women who had removal of the uterus but still have ovaries. I certainly find these same objective confirmations in my evaluations of hormone levels.

How can women become prematurely menopausal after a hysterectomy? The uterine artery has to be "tied off" (clamped) when the uterus is removed. Otherwise, you would have uncontrollable bleeding. When this artery is tied off, it means a loss of over 50% of the blood flow to the ovary from the uterine artery. The ovary still gets some blood flow from another, smaller artery in the wall of the pelvis, but this does not make up for what is lost from the uterine artery. You can imagine how difficult it is for the ovary to function to make its hormones if it only has *half* it's normal blood supply.

2. Doctors tell women with *one* ovary removed, "Don't worry, the other ovary will take over and make enough hormones. You'll be fine." Try telling *that* to a man who has lost one testicle. *One* ovary does not typically do the job of two.

3. Even after complete removal of both ovaries with the uterus, causing instant menopause, with estrogen levels plunging lower than a man's, and loss of about 90% of our testosterone, only about 25-30% of women start hormone therapy. Only about half of those women take it for longer than 5 years. This means a huge number of women with *no ovaries* are going without any replacement of the very hormones needed for a myriad of body and brain systems. I don't believe it is just the loss of the uterus that causes so many health problems, including loss of sexual function. I think a bigger overlooked issue is the loss of our ovarian hormones that play crucial metabolic roles throughout our body—from sex to weight to energy level to memory and mood and sleep and pain regulation, to name just a few.

4. Even if women *do* start hormone therapy after a hysterectomy, most still do not get "optimal" replacement of their ovarian hormones. The usual approach is to simply give estrogen, usually Premarin, a mixture of horse-derived estrogens foreign to our bodies that provides very little of the 17beta-estradiol our bodies have always made, and need. Testosterone is rarely replaced. Testosterone enhances energy level, libido, sense of well being and mood, bone and muscle formation and also (along with estradiol) improves the vaginal tissue to relieve dryness that causes pain during sex. Even though medical studies going back to the 1950s show the benefits, and safety, of testosterone replacement, the vast majority who have had hysterectomy *still* are not offered testosterone therapy. And hormone levels are rarely checked; there is typically no individualization of type, route, or dose of estrogen. It doesn't have to be this way. I work hard to help my

patients achieve optimal hormone replacement, and most are amazed at the degree of well being that can return with the right type of hormone replacement, the right delivery approach, and optimal levels.

5. Depression following hysterectomy is assumed to be psychological reaction to losing the uterus. Dr. Studd's view, which is confirmed by my own clinical experience, is that "a more plausible cause of depression is the varying degree of ovarian hormone deficiency, which is often overlooked and untreated following hysterectomy." I certainly agree; clinical experience and a number of research studies show that depressed moods, low energy, sleep loss, anxiety, and loss of libido *can be* alleviated with good hormone management. A long-term prospective study published in 1992 found no depression at four months after hysterectomy, but depression did develop after 24 months, which supports that depression is not likely just from an emotional reaction to hysterectomy but can occur as the ovarian hormones decline overtime. Such a gradual decrease in estradiol and testosterone just may not produce *noticeable* symptoms for two or more years after the surgery.

What does this mean for you? If you are only 30 years old and have a hysterectomy, even if you keep both ovaries, you have a 30-60% chance of having *menopausal* hormone levels within three years of the surgery though you are still in your thirties. In fact, even when your ovaries work well for many years, studies show that you will become menopausal about 4 to 5 years earlier than average. But if no one is checking your hormone levels with reliable blood tests, the hormone cause of symptoms is missed. Fatigue, headaches, depression, insomnia, loss of sex drive, and other symptoms are more likely labeled depression, chronic fatigue, anxiety, or stress.

6. The hormone furor of 2002, with major headlines screaming the dangers of "estrogen" based on studies (HERS, WHI, in particular) using only Prempro—the horse-derived estrogen and synthetic progestin has unnecessarily frightened many women into being afraid of taking "hormones" after hysterectomy. Yet what is overlooked is that this product is *not* our natural estrogen, and it is a mixture of a potent synthetic progestin that itself can have many negative effects. In the Women's Health Initiative (WHI) study, the estrogen-only group (women who had previously had hysterectomy) was not stopped because this group was not showing the negative outcomes found in the Prempro group. The media seemed to ignore this crucial point. There is *good* news about the emerging research showing many benefits of the ovary's natural estradiol—and testosterone—for many dimensions of women's well being and health. The media also ignores crucial difference between the synthetic progestin used in the WHI and the natural ovarian hormone, progesterone, which often has fewer adverse side effects. Sadly, such positive findings often don't get reported in the media that seems to focus on sensationalizing the negative and promoting fear.

7. In view of the points I made above, I encourage women to consider carefully the pros and cons of removing the ovaries at the time of hysterectomy. Many of the 450,000 annual "prophylactic" oophorectomies may not really be necessary if women have healthy ovaries and no family history or risk factors for ovarian cancer. For other women, removal of the ovaries may be necessary because of a high risk of ovarian cancer, recurrent painful cysts, or endometriomas, and adhesions, to name a few. In addition, many women don't realize that severe, intractable PMS can persist, and may even worsen, if the ovaries are left in because ovarian cycles continue, even without the uterus. But for younger women without these problems, there may be many reasons to leave the ovaries so natural hormone

production can continue. Just remember to have your levels checked with reliable blood tests if you start having symptoms that suggest hormone decline.

Having a hysterectomy doesn't *have* to inevitably mean loss of one's quality of life. I know there is a better way to prevent such disastrous outcomes that rob women of their sexuality, their sense of womanhood, and their body-mind-spirit health. If you have spent years suffering, not feeling well, and going from doctor to doctor trying to find a way to relieve symptoms and to feel better, start your journey to regaining your well being by insisting on having your hormone levels properly checked with today's "gold standard" blood tests! It is not difficult or overly expensive to do. Then read about the many options, life-style choices, and complementary approaches to help you regain hormone balance and health. You deserve to have your health concerns taken seriously.

—Elizabeth Lee Vliet, M.D.
> Author of *It's My OVARIES, Stupid!; Women, Weight and Hormones; Screaming to Be Heard: Hormone Connections Women Suspect and Doctors Still Ignore*
> Founder and Medical Director, HER Place: Health Enhancement and Renewal for Women, Inc. - Tucson, Arizona

Personal Notes

Hysterectomy Only

Writer's Profile

ഗ3ഗ3ഗ3ഗ3ഗ3ഗ3ഗ3ഗ3ഗ3ഗ3 ಜುಜುಜುಜುಜುಜುಜುಜುಜುಜು

Authored by: Charis Wilson

Age: 39

From: Denver, CO USA

Hysterectomy: 1999

Age at surgery 36

Ovary removed No

Age at surgery N/A

Reason for
surgery/surgeries: Endometriosis, dysmenorrhea,
and extreme cramping

Hormone replacement
history: None

Other medications: None

I should start by saying I was one of the lucky ones who had a doctor who not only encouraged me to do my own research before making any decision, but expected it. She also encouraged me to bring along a friend, in my case my mother, during my pre-surgical consultation. She willingly answered my questions as well as my mother's.

I had reached the point of considering a hysterectomy after more than two decades of trying to cure or treat my endometriosis, disabling cramping, and dysmenorrhea. Every month saw me heavily bleeding for two weeks. I was constantly anemic and had cramps that would have knocked a horse over. My life had reached the point where I planned everything, both personally and professionally, around my periods. In fact, I had reached a point where I had no life, I couldn't do the things I enjoyed.

Over the years, a score of doctors had tried treating me with a variety of birth control formulas, all with no success. Several doctors, including a couple of women, told me that there was nothing wrong with me and that it was all in my head. Then I got lucky and found a doctor that could help me.

I found her through an advertisement in the local paper for a study she was conducting on endometrial ablation. I had read several articles on this new procedure and knew it was being used to successfully treat excessive bleeding like mine. After my first consultation, during which she assured me that bleeding like mine was not normal and was not all in my head, she scheduled me for a series of tests. In the meantime, she had me keep a sanitary supply diary during my next three periods.

Unfortunately the tests revealed that I was not a good candidate for the ablation procedure. My doctor, though, did not abandon me. She continued to treat my condition. We tried several other drugs and a hysteroscopy D&C. However nothing worked, and in December of 1998 she informed me that the only option left was a hysterectomy.

Being a librarian, I am a firm believer in the adage that knowledge is power, so I read everything I could get my hands on regarding hysterectomy. Based upon that research, I went into my pre-surgery consultation with a list of about twenty questions, all of which the doctor answered. I elected to have a sub-total hysterectomy (cervix left in place), and the doctor agreed that she would not remove my ovaries. Moreover, she agreed that if during the surgery she determined that it would be medically necessary to remove either of my ovaries, she would consult with my mother first before actually doing so.

It turned out that she did not need to remove either of my ovaries, although she did warn me that one of them was so scarred from the endometriosis that it will likely shut down on its own in about five years. It was also lucky that we had already decided to leave my cervix in, as it had fused to my rectum from the endometriosis scarring.

It has now been almost two years since my surgery and I'm literally a new woman. I no longer have to plan my days around the proximity of a toilet. I am no longer suffering from permanent anemia. I have my life back. I can now travel and indulge in my passion for hot air ballooning. In fact, earlier this year I bought my own balloon and am now learning to fly it, something I could not have done before since balloon rides meant being more than fifty feet away from a toilet. I will be eternally grateful to my doctor for saving my life, by giving my life back to me.

—Charis Wilson - Denver, CO USA

Writer's Profile

ೞೞೞೞೞೞೞೞೞೞೞ   ೞೞೞೞೞೞೞೞೞೞ

Authored by:	Laurie
Age:	46
From:	Puyallup, Washington USA
Hysterectomy:	1994
Age at surgery	38
Ovary removed	No
Age at surgery	N/A
Reason for surgery/surgeries:	Fibroids
Hormone replacement history:	Not reported
Other medications:	Not reported

When I was 38, I began to have problems with heavy bleeding. At the time, I went to my family doctor and she prescribed birth control pills to control the bleeding. My husband had a vasectomy, so I certainly didn't need them to prevent pregnancy! The pill slowed the bleeding, but also caused me to gain 15 pounds in a month. So my doctor referred me to a gynecologist, who performed an ultrasound and discovered fibroid tumors in my uterus. Naturally, he prescribed a hysterectomy. It sounded good to me; my family was complete, no more periods!

In the hospital, the day of the surgery, the nurse handed me an informational booklet about the procedure. It was very slick, in color, obviously printed and handed out for the occasion. It said, "Your life will not change at all because of your surgery. You can go on with your life exactly as before, ESPECIALLY YOUR SEX LIFE. Your body and responses will be exactly the same as before, without the inconvenience and pain of periods."

The thing is, I was not the type to buy everything the medical establishment feeds us. I've always questioned unnecessary medical practices. I delivered both my babies with midwives, the second one at home. However, I could find no negative information about hysterectomy, so I went into the operation totally believing it would be a good thing for me.

The first thing I noticed, about three weeks after the surgery, was a pronounced constipation.[1] I've always been healthy and athletic, with a high fiber, low fat, semi-vegetarian diet. This was not just normal constipation, but was an absolute absence of normal physical urge to have a bowel movement! I searched the library for information, with no results. To this day, the process of bowel movements is very painful, and still not normal for me. I asked my gynecologist about it at my second post-surgery visit, and his reaction was vehement denial that the operation had anything to do with my problem. I've tried to be accepting and philosophical about it, but it does cause me a lot of physical discomfort. I e-mailed the National Digestive Diseases Information Clearinghouse about this. They had no information on the relation of hysterectomy to irritable bowel syndrome (IBS).[1]

The second thing I noticed after surgery was a pronounced reduction in the intensity of my orgasms.[2] I've always had a satisfying sexual relationship with my husband of 20 years. I also know how to facilitate my own orgasms. A few months after the surgery, I realized things were not getting back to normal. The response is about half of what it used to be, and we've tried every trick in the book. I'm almost positive this is not a psychological response, but a physical one. How can the uterus NOT play a major response in the muscular response of orgasm?

They took my cervix, but not my ovaries. I still feel hormonal changes every month, such as breast tenderness and skin break outs, so I don't think my ovaries have shut down. I feel that this reduction of orgasmic response is hysterectomized women's "dirty little secret" that no one wants to talk about.

I guess I don't totally regret the operation; as young as I was, I probably would have had to go back for a second surgery if I'd only had a myomectomy. I just wish I'd been more informed, so I would have had some idea what to expect.

—Laurie - Puyallup, Washington USA

Writer's Profile

ଓଓଓଓଓଓଓଓଓଓଓଓ ଐଐଐଐଐଐଐଐଐଐ

Authored by: KDeit
Age: 56
From: Kissimmee, Florida USA

Hysterectomy: 2001
Age at surgery   55

Ovary removed   No
Age at surgery   N/A

Reason for
    surgery/surgeries: Prolapses of uterus, bowel and
                          bladder

Hormone replacement
    history: 1998 to present
                          Prempro™ 1998 to 2001
                          Premarin® 2001 to 2002
                          Estradiol 2002 to present

Other medications: Fosamax® (low bone density),
                        Prevacid® and gaviscon (acid
                        reflux)

I was eleven when I started my periods. They were so painful that I missed a couple of days of school almost every month until a doctor finally put me on birth control pills, which did help lessen the pain. I went off of them in order to have my two children, and each time found that my periods were very painful when I wasn't on the pill.

However, I was also a smoker, and when I turned 35 my doctor refused to continue to prescribe the pill unless I quit. I wasn't ready to stop smoking at that time, and so I put up with the painful periods in order to smoke (looking back on it now, I can't believe I made that choice!). It turned out that most of my pain was caused by mild endometriosis, which was removed during a laparoscopy, and did not come back. Then, about ten years ago, my doctor told me that I could either quit smoking, or I could look forward to a future of dragging an oxygen tank around with me. That finally woke me up, and I went to a psychologist who uses hypnosis. I had two sessions with him and threw my cigarettes away!

Then, about five years ago, I began to have symptoms of menopause. I had heavy bleeding, night sweats, hot flashes, and mood swings (cried at any and everything) so badly that after a year or so, my husband asked me to please go to a doctor and get something to make me feel better. I did, and took Prempro for a few years, which helped until my uterus began to prolapse. I tried Kegel exercises for about 18 months, but eventually it got to the point that I felt as if everything was falling out. In addition, it turned out that I also had a rectocele and a cystocele, along with the uterine prolapse. I was scheduled for a vaginal hysterectomy along with anterior and posterior repairs for the cystocele and rectocele in August 2001. My doctor was very uncommunicative and I didn't know the questions that I should have asked, nor did I know at all what to expect.

The night before my surgery, when I was so nervous that I couldn't sleep, I sat down at the computer and typed in "hysterectomy." Well, I found a hysterectomy Website where I immediately felt as if I'd found a whole new family. I only wish that I had found it earlier than I did.

My surgery was scheduled for 6:30 AM and it went quite well—I had general anesthesia, and had absolutely no side effects from it at all. I woke up around noon in my room, hooked up to a morphine pump. My family and the nurse tell me that I never let the controller button out of my fist all morning, but I have no recollection of any pain or discomfort at all. The next morning the nurses removed my catheter and the gauze packing that was inside my vagina. Removing it was not painful, but it was a strange feeling, and it seemed to take forever before it was all out.

I was released in the early afternoon, the day after my surgery, and was sent home with a prescription for Percocet. The ride home was quite uncomfortable, because I didn't realize how painful the rectocele and cystocele incisions would be, and had not thought to bring a donut pillow to sit on. In fact, I didn't have one until two or three days later, when I asked my daughter to buy me one, after reading that suggestion on the hysterectomy Website. After that, it was a lot easier to sit, although I was still very uncomfortable for several more weeks from the episiotomy–like incisions.

I began to itch terribly after I'd been home for just a few days (I didn't realize that it might be an allergic reaction to the Percocet). I finally called my doctor and she prescribed Darvocet, which was not quite as strong, but it relieved the itching.

I was also given a prescription for Premarin (1.25 mg), which I started right away. I began to have a lot of vaginal discharge, which was not something I had prior to my hysterectomy, and it turned out that the Premarin dosage was too high for me. After some trial-and-error, I ended up on 0.625 mg, which I continued to take until two weeks ago. Recently, I had read about bio-identical estrogen on the hysterectomy Website, and I am now taking 1 mg of estradiol instead. So far, I'm having no problems with the estradiol, but it's only been two weeks, which is too soon to know if I will be able to continue on it or not.

I was released to go back to work 5 1/2 weeks after my hysterectomy, and did, but I probably should have started back part-time for the first couple of weeks instead of full-time. I was totally worn out by the time I got home at night, and if my husband hadn't been willing to cook, we would have eaten a lot of fast foods those first few weeks.

I was cleared to resume sexual relations at six weeks after surgery, but found that it was too painful, so we waited a couple of weeks longer. At first we had to use quite a bit of lubricant, since the repairs made things quite a bit tighter. Now that I am 17 months postoperative and completely healed, I have found that, if anything, sex is better than it was before my hysterectomy.[2] It is no longer painful.

Finally, I want to thank you for your goal of encouraging the medical community to do more research on women's issues and finding answers for our problems.

—KDeit - Kissimmee, Florida USA

Writer's Profile

ෲෲෲෲෲෲෲෲෲෲ   🍒   ෲෲෲෲෲෲෲෲෲෲ

Authored by:	Nina
Age:	39
From:	Indiana USA
Hysterectomy:	2001
Age at surgery	37
Ovary removed	No
Age at surgery	N/A
Reason for surgery/surgeries:	Recurrent cervical dysplasia and vaginal carcinoma-in-situ (precancer condition of cervix and vaginal wall)
Hormone replacement history:	None
Other medications:	None

My history of gynecologic problems started in 1987, when I was 23 years old. I had just given birth to my first child and my six-week follow-up Pap smear came back showing severe dysplasia. I was treated with a cone biopsy and was told that for 90% of women, that was all the treatment that was needed. I was part of that 90% group for almost ten years.

Four more children later, in 1996, I was diagnosed with moderate dysplasia and was treated with cryotherapy (cold used to destroy abnormal cells). In 1998, after one more child, I was diagnosed with moderate dysplasia and treated with cryotherapy again. During that time, I also developed a vaginal tear that would reopen during intercourse or with internal exams. It got progressively worse over time, to the point that intercourse really was not an option. In December of 2000, I had another abnormal Pap and my doctor and I agreed to pursue a LEEP (loop electrocautery excision procedure) and D&C for further diagnostic work and, hopefully, treatment for the condition. I requested that he repair the vaginal tear at the same time. The pathology was somewhat surprising to me. The cervical biopsy showed moderate dysplasia, and the vaginal biopsy showed carcinoma-in-situ with no clear margins (precancer not all removed).

A hysterectomy was recommended due to my lengthy history of recurrences and because of all the scar tissue from the previous procedures, which made it difficult to get quality cells for examination. Essentially, I could have cancerous cells and no one would know it because there weren't enough good-quality cells to examine. It was also suggested that a larger vaginal resection (vagina cut and resewn) be completed to try to remove the rest of the abnormal cells on the vaginal wall.

It was with a heavy heart and many tears that I agreed to go forward with the hysterectomy. I was terrified! I was afraid that if I did not have the surgery that my condition would eventually become cancerous, and I would not be around to see my children graduate from high school. Almost as bad, I was afraid of losing my identity as a woman. I had read all the horror stories about women regretting their decisions. They had chronic pain, bladder problems, hormone issues, depression, loss of libido (sex drive)—the list went on and on. Still, I felt I had no choice. I immediately began mourning the future loss of orgasms and desire for intimacy, and went into surgery.

I had a total abdominal hysterectomy, which was completed in just under three hours. There were a few adhesions from my previous C-sections and some mild endometriosis (I had been having some mild symptoms of this, but had not really recognized it at the time). A vaginal resection was also completed. I was able to keep my healthy ovaries, so I did not require hormone replacement. I was discharged within days feeling very sore, tired, sad, and alone. It was difficult and uncomfortable to move about with both an abdominal and a vaginal incision. About ten days after surgery, I had the worst yeast infection I have ever had. It completely covered my perineal region from pubic bone to tail bone. I was miserable, and still sad.

I started to surf the web for short periods of time looking for answers. I struck it rich one day and found a hysterectomy support group on the Internet. What a place! It was loaded with information and stories and support. Even better, it was totally run by women who were going through the same thing I was going through. It was like I had found a whole new circle of friends, and all of them understood my fears and concerns. I found a wonderful forum there, which addresses the specific issues of women diagnosed with various gynecologic cancers and precancers. I also found hope that my life would return to normal—there is life after a hysterectomy.

I healed well. I had several rounds of bacterial vaginosis (vaginal infections) followed by yeast infections. I could not seem to get my body chemistry back in order. It was very frustrating! I was very tired for the first six months, but that gradually improved, and now, two years after my surgery, I can honestly say that my energy level is similar to that before my surgery, although I do require an extra hour of sleep every night. I feel very much like my previous self—keeping my ovaries helped. My hormones continue to cycle just as they did before my surgery, so my internal clock continues to work. It was more than a year before I could comfortably have intercourse again. My vaginal area was sore and swollen for a long time from the extensive work. It was a physically painful and emotionally difficult time, but it was made easier by the love and support I found at my hysterectomy Internet support group. My husband and family were also wonderfully supportive, but I found it easier to discuss the very intimate details of my recovery with my "cyber-sisters."

I had one abnormal Pap approximately one year after surgery, but all others have been normal. I am still afraid that the abnormal cells will return someplace on my vaginal wall, and I have Pap's completed every three months to watch for this. All of this has made me so much more aware of my general health status. I am eating a healthier diet, getting better sleep, exercising more regularly, taking appropriate vitamin supplements, and practicing yoga. I am doing what I can to strengthen my immune system in hopes of keeping a recurrence at bay. I am also keeping my fingers crossed that researchers will soon find a way to deal with this virus (human papillomavirus), which is known to contribute to the development of most cases of cervical cancer. Millions of women carry some form of this virus. Fortunately, most never have any symptoms or problems, but it is a huge health concern for all of us and for our daughters in the future.

I have come to believe that a gynecologist is the most important member of a woman's health care team. My gynecologist has been wonderful throughout this ordeal. He has been open and honest, caring, encouraging, and diligent in his efforts to get all of the information I needed to make the right choices for me.

—Nina - Indiana USA

Writer's Profile

CECECECECECECECECE ຽວຽວຽວຽວຽວຽວຽວຽວ

Authored by:	"Falling Out"
Age:	51
From:	Washington USA
Hysterectomy:	2001
Age at surgery	50
Ovary removed	No
Age at surgery	N/A
Reason for surgery/surgeries:	3rd degree rectocele, and 2nd degree uterine prolapse
Hormone replacement history:	2001 (on and off) Estropipate
Other medications:	Not reported

I thought the best way to tell of my experience was to utilize the progression of my hysterectomy experience through the letters that I wrote to all my care givers. It has been instructive for me to go back and reread them, as I realize how little I knew when I made such a big decision. At the time, I couldn't even spell the medical terms right. Now I know much more about the terms, my physical body, and the functioning of health care systems.

November 13, 2001—Letter to my surgeon:

Dear Doctor:

I am one of your patients who had a hysterectomy and rectocele repairs about two months ago, and experienced three weeks of intense vaginal itching. Since my six-week post-op visit, I've had an epiphany of sorts, which might have some bearing on how you could treat others with the same problem.

When I was barely pregnant with my first child, my body suddenly looked like a war zone, and I had intolerable itching. The doctors had me wrap up in wet sheets for a couple of days while they tried to figure out what was up (one doctor suggested mites—and thought I should rub my entire body in Vaseline). When I went in the second day for another look, a dermatologist came in who took one look at me, pulled out a tongue depressor, and swiped it across my back. Then I heard a collective "Ohhhh" behind me. It turned out that somehow the hormonal surge of pregnancy had given me a weird dermatological response, such that even a tongue depressor swipe could make my skin welt. At any rate, after they convinced me that only if I buried myself in Benadryl could it hurt my baby, I took it, got a good night sleep, and woke up still looking horrible, but feeling fine. If a tongue depressor could welt my back under the right conditions, seems logical to me that a knife and stitches could do wild things to a vagina. Although not an allergy in a medical sense, something was making an intense abnormal reaction. So perhaps something as simple as Benadryl could have broken that itch cycle. It wouldn't have hurt anything—and at the very least I could have had a decent nights sleep without disturbing dreams. As I recall, Benadryl was first marketed as a sleep aid for the insane—which is close to what I felt! It's too bad I didn't think of that—but I was probably too busy visualizing some hidden necrotic sore, trying desperately to distract myself by keeping busy, or coming up with bizarre coping methods involving tea tree oil and fans . . . .

I was upset that I had to call, call, and call, and finally throw a hissy fit after a week in order to be seen by anyone. Although you assured me that all was fine, continued itching led me to close self-examination, which unfortunately just gave me new fears. I realized that no one could see what was going on in there—the opening was so pitifully tiny. So now I not only felt itchy and scared, but also profoundly sad, angry, and ruined. I turned to the Internet to figure out just what I had done to myself—and what more I might expect. At least I could get some comfort about the things that didn't happen—for example, at least I wasn't dead.

While it's understandable that doctors with patients they know well may be able to diagnose and prescribe things over the phone, I was uncomfortable being diagnosed with a yeast infection, especially since to my knowledge I've never had one.

The good news is, I'm feeling much better. The rectocele symptoms that I had in the post-op visit are gone, and I now only have general aches, and momentary pain. I have some residual itch; sort of a tickle, but it's not bothersome. Some people have phantom limbs—maybe I have a phantom uterus . . . . At any rate, it responds well to "scratching." I am sexually responsive, but we do have to do things differently. I can run now, have no lower back pain, and I found out I lost seven pounds (nothing like weeks of terror to take off weight). I'm bleeding much less, just two mini-pads per day.

I got the impression during my post-op visit that you were quite satisfied with the surgical side of my healing, but you suggested another visit to placate me. Since I'm feeling physically fine, I've cancelled that visit—so you can note the above paragraph in my chart and mark me down for the most part as a surgical success. Case closed. It's too bad my post-op experience was so traumatic. In time it will make a funny story, but right now I'm still a little shaky. I never quite grasped how terrified I had been until things started working okay again.

Now I'll turn my thoughts to more exciting things—like preparing for our backpacking trip to the wilds of Honduras next month.

Sincerely,

February 1, 2002 — Next is a letter 4 1/2 months post-op, where I'm still trying hard to recover—but realize I'm just not . . .

Dear Doctor:

You performed my hysterectomy for prolapse 4 1/2 months ago. I wrote to you after my postoperative examination, saying that I was just fine—which I wanted very much to be. At the time, I was both physically and emotionally shaken and did not want to go back. I just wanted the entire experience to go away. The statement that I was doing fine was premature, and some functioning that I had anticipated has not returned. Thus, I need to clarify for my record to state that in my view, the surgery has not been successful.

For the past 2 1/2 months, I have tried three different times to resume my running routine, which is running three miles every other day. I would find that after gradually working up to this for a week, I would have to stop, since I began feeling like things in my pelvic area were dropping. I know that lifting weights like I used to would not be a good idea, especially since just lifting groceries puts pressure there. So recently, I decided to resume yoga again, to continue to keep up my strength while waiting to try running again. However, in certain poses I actually feel like I am splitting apart. This is not low pain—which pelvic floor exercises help—it is a high, jabbing pain. This is not a pain I can "work through," as the intensity makes me collapse. Before surgery, you had discussed how some women might need to have further surgery after hysterectomy for prolapse, but this is not an option for me. My vagina has widened over time, but has not lengthened. Although sex is good, my husband has to avoid certain positions for thrusting or it becomes painful.[2] Any further repairs could significantly impair my sexual functioning. While I suppose if men can be changed into women, it is technically feasible to rebuild my vagina by using skin grafts and Gore-Tex or whatnot, however this is obviously not desirable.

I am discouraged. Before surgery, there was discomfort when running at times and with other activities, but I always felt that things could be "fixed." Now, I feel afraid to do the things I always loved doing, for fear I will do more irreparable damage. Before surgery, I had been able to read my body signals, and recovered from things well. That hasn't been the case this time. I feel very foolish that I had this operation. I was hoping for a better quality of life, not restrictions. Perhaps I was too young. If I had been older, and had the opportunity to gradually and naturally slow down, maybe I wouldn't notice being so physically limited. It is like I've instantly aged 15 years.

So from my point of view, I would not classify the surgery as successful. While I will still be able to enjoy life—I was doing that before surgery—without as many fears or restrictions. Is there anything more I can do, or is this just "me"?

Sincerely,

March 25, 2002 — The next letter I wrote to all the people I had dealt with at the surgical group, and to my family doctor and nurse practitioner.

Dear Doctors and Nurse,

Your office performed my hysterectomy for prolapse and rectocele six months ago, and I am disturbed at the way I was treated. Understanding how bad my pre- and postoperative care was might spur change in the ways you do things so others will not have to suffer needlessly. It would have taken only a few more moments to give proper care, and I would have been reassured that the physicians knew what they were doing. My concerns are in the following areas:

1.   Proper Assessment. After my operation, I read literature written by doctors to help decide about surgery options. A major theme is the importance of proper assessment. Each section of the vagina—anterior, posterior, lateral, and apex—must be inspected and evaluated separately to define the true nature and degree of prolapse. If prolapse is present in one place, there may be weakness in another. Diagnosing these correctly directly affects surgical success. Some physicians have patients fill out sheets that document problems, or ask questions. The literature explained physical tests that doctors might likely give you, and questions they would ask. A good summary of this literature is found in: "Pelvic Prolapse: Diagnosis & Treating Cystoceles, Rectoceles & Enteroceles" Cespedes et al, *Medscape Women's Health eJournal*, 3(4) 1998. I received very limited tests or questions. Perhaps there is a school of thought that advocates a "cut and see" approach, but I didn't read about that anywhere. After my operation you asked: "You didn't have any problems with your bladder, did you?" Too woozy to be concerned then—now that I understand the importance of proper diagnosis—I wonder if I was properly assessed.

2.   Postoperative Care. I experienced intense itching. Without an exam, the nurse prescribed medicine for a yeast infection over the phone. I explained that I do not get yeast infections. The medication provided no relief. Several phone calls and a week later, I was able to get an appointment to be seen. When I arrived, I was told that I couldn't be seen. I insisted—and was finally seen by the doctor. He told me I was fine. He suggested I use cortisone cream, and tested for yeast infection, for which I had already been unnecessarily treated. He said that my surgeon would not be available. I had to endure the same intense itching for two more weeks. Itching like poison ivy in your vagina and genitals is terrible. It seemed systemic (body wide), affecting my nervous system, and thinking processes, as well as my vagina.

I thought I was right to insist upon being seen. I had extensive surgical repairs after my first child was born, and my doctor at the time told me I should have come in before my six-week scheduled visit, since my stitches were infected, and he could have helped. I did not feel as bad with that infection as I did with what I experienced after my hysterectomy. I also discovered in my reading that medical groups who test for yeast infection after hysterectomies have found that women rarely have them—that the postoperative intense itching is due to something else.

3.   Lack of Trust and Communication. At my post-op exam, my surgeon was not interested in my concern about the intense reaction, which had been troubling me for three weeks, choosing instead to say, "I'm sorry if I did not tell you that you had a major operation." This response made me feel that I had been a nuisance. No one can advocate properly for themselves when distressed and vulnerable. I left confused, thinking I was considered a bad patient because I was not healing well. He said we could meet in another month, suggesting that I could then tell him what he should tell other women the next time he operated. I

felt patronized, and that my problems were not being addressed. I was not confident with the seriousness with which my problems would be addressed, so did not return. I sought help at my primary care physician's office.

4.   Duration of Recovery Time. I scheduled my operation three months before an active vacation. Friends who had had hysterectomies, and even medical doctors assured me that time frame was sufficient—even if something went wrong. Not so! When I flew off for vacation, I was sore, had stopped bleeding only three days before, felt like a golf ball was in my rectum, had to physically hold up my anus with my fingers for a bowel movement, was unable to carry my own backpack, and was not up for any strenuous hiking. If I had been comfortable with visiting the surgeon, perhaps he could have allayed my fears and explained that these symptoms would not last.

5.   Options. If I had been aware that less invasive options to rectocele and prolapse repair are available through laparoscopy, either with or without removing the uterus, I would have explored them. This procedure allows women to preserve the integrity of their vagina with minimal scarring. Many physicians think it is unnecessary to remove a uterus for prolapse unless diseased (literature from numerous physicians of the Society of Gynecologic Surgeons). I did not read about such procedures until after my surgery, when trying to diagnose my physical problems. At 4 1/2 months post-op, I still was not healed, but was strong enough to go back to my surgeon. I realized that only a gynecologist could address the questions and problems that I had, such as concerns that my vagina was too short now for any future repair options. He did not mention those options then, either.

While even good surgeons can have bad luck, I am left wondering after my surgery: whether I was assessed properly;

when the surgeon last preformed the kind of surgery that I had; whether all his patients take twice as long as normal to heal; or when the staff last examined current medical literature?

I realize now that surgeons who want to know your symptoms and take the time to properly assess your specific problems before surgery, will probably also want to know about any postoperative reactions to help assess problems, ease discomfort, and allay fears afterwards. Patients should not have to be "strong enough" to visit a doctor. Physicians are supposed to aid sick and vulnerable clients. The surgical experience I had may have been the norm for my mother's generation—but it is not adequate enough for mine.

I am hoping this letter will spur a reassessment of your pre- and postoperative procedures and reevaluation of your approach to surgery and patient care. If it could spare some other unsuspecting victim, I mean patient, then it will be well worth it.

Sincerely,

June 13, 2002 — I was finally able to go to another gynecologist, who labeled my surgery as "an expensive mistake," and told me to send the above letter to the head of my HMO (Health Maintenance Organization). This is the letter I wrote to him:

Dear Medical Director,

I visited a doctor in your HMO for a consult last Tuesday, June 12, 2002 regarding complications from a hysterectomy performed on September 18, 2001. At his recommendation, I am sending the letter of concern to you that I had sent on March 25, 2002 to the gynecological group who performed my surgery.

I have had problems with my bowels since surgery,[1] and have developed urge incontinence within the last two months.[3] I had physical therapy for incontinence before surgery to try to avoid surgery. I will be setting up appointments to see a urologist about urge incontinence, and another specialist about the problems with my bowels, which he suspects may be due to nerve damage from surgery.

I have been frustrated navigating through your HMO system. While the literature states that it is a state law that women can self refer to a gynecologist, your organization does not provide any information about your doctors' qualifications so that women can choose the best doctor for their problems. Patients must rely on their family doctors for referrals, or "hope" that the gynecologist they go to will refer them to another doctor with more experience and expertise. In my case, this presented a problem. I was referred to a gynecologist who I now suspect did not have the proper qualifications to address my problems, and did not refer me to a specialist who was qualified to manage my needs. As a result, I am experiencing unsatisfactory results. I suggest that your organization make information on physicians available to your patients, as they do in other clinics. Had I known that this was available, I would have requested it at the outset.

I would also recommend that patients with prolapse be required to see an expert before surgery, to ensure that they are properly assessed, and to determine if surgery can fix their problems. It is a terrible expense for your organization, as well as a terrible experience for the patient to have unnecessary surgery, or surgery that does not work.

Sincerely,

June 28, 2002 — The next letter I wrote to the head of the HMO again—after I had the opportunity to read my surgeon's notes and realized they were nutty!

Dear Doctor:

Thank you for reviewing my case. To better understand what happened to me, I recently reviewed my surgeon's notes, and thought I should bring some things to your attention.

In reading the reports from the surgeon, there are some errors. One notable one is the statement: "Patient denies urinary incontinence." I do not know whether you will ask for the reports from my physical therapist or family doctor, but I have enclosed the final physical therapy report, which clearly shows that I would never deny urinary incontinence. One would presume that this report would have been forwarded to the surgeon.

Also, I am enclosing two other letters I sent to the surgeon. The first, dated November 13, 2001, while poorly written and thought out, it accurately portrays a patient in shock, trying to understand and make the best of a traumatic event. The second, dated February 1, 2002, asks for advice and details specific problems.

While patient care was certainly sub par in my case, the larger, and more important issue is the lack of continuing training and education of the physicians. While I am not a doctor, from my subsequent reading and from my consult, I think that there needs to be an education effort to address exactly what can and cannot be remedied by performing a hysterectomy, so that unnecessary hysterectomies, like mine may have been, can be avoided.

Sincerely,

September 28, 2002 — The last letter is to my family doctor when I switched doctors.

Dear Doctor:

It has been a year since my surgery for prolapse and rectocele, and I think it is instructive for you to know of the outcome up to now. I hope that this letter will help ensure that no other woman in your practice will experience such a horrible experience. I have seen an oncologist/gynecologist who has had specific training in pelvic floor repairs, a urologist, a colorectal specialist, had a defogram performed, and have seen a urogynecologist.

I have been diagnosed with a "mild to moderate" cystocele, which is what gives me the feeling that my vagina is falling out when going to the bathroom. Fortunately, my incontinence is not presently related to that, and can be handled for now by continued physical therapy, diet, and medication that has been prescribed for it. This will need to be monitored since future surgery will probably be necessary.

The colorectal specialist found a rectocele, which had been presenting problems. He sent me for a defogram, which confirms the diagnosis. He considered my case complicated, and referred me to the urogynecologist. She could not see the rectocele through my vagina, but noted that I now have symptoms of rectal prolapse and some muscular problems for which I will have therapy. She also found my vagina short with much scarring, which would make further surgery tricky. She does not do that type of surgery, but there are physicians who do (I have become a more knowledgable consumer and ask about their expertise before surgery—not after).

After extensive research I now recognize my nightmare may never end—that when prolapse problems are not addressed properly initially, they may never be resolved, but I am hopeful that things can be better.

This should not have happened. I have some suggestions to prevent your patients from being ruined by out of date and careless gynecologists:

1.   Promote patient education.
2.   Promote obtaining second opinions.
3.   Check out the credentials of the surgeons.
4.   Suggest that your patients read surgeon's charts before the operation. I was shocked to find strange things in my charts eight months after the surgery. The most shocking was an indented statement in the middle of a block that says, "Patient denies urinary incontinence." I wrote the day after he examined me that he said, "You must feel that you need to go to the bathroom all the time!" He also told me that so much was falling down that nothing short of surgery could ever hold it up. This is classic bamboozle that surgeons use to get women to have hysterectomies—who knows why in my notes he wrote I denied urinary incontinence. Hard to believe I was so trusting. Like a bad scientist who does an experiment then writes his hypothesis, perhaps he performed the operation then wrote his notes. It makes me sick to think of a physician in that way. I wonder at the integrity of the surgical notes. What "surprises" will another surgeon find when they try to re-repair me?

It is a frustrating experience to instinctively know that something is wrong medically, but have physicians trivialize or not pursue the problems. By the time I saw another doctor, I was confused and frightened by the symptoms, and frantically trying to figure things out on my own. The new staff were all excellent, compassionate, and like good detectives helped me sort through the symptoms, and methodically addressed them. No one made me feel that my problems were non-existent or trivial. This is the type of gynecological care that I was used to.

It is important to note that before surgery, although I felt heaviness in my pelvic area that was very annoying, I had no noticeable cystocele. I had a sensation of incomplete bowel movement, but no problems evacuating my bowels. Now, I have painful bowel movements that I can only have while standing up. My entire anus becomes purple and swollen when I defecate, and if I sit down and try holding it up, I occasionally spurt blood. The colorectal specialist says it is not a hemorrhoid. In reviewing my surgery, I think the only successful procedure was the removal of the uterus, which still feels like it was removed by a chain saw. However, it may not have been necessary, and may have contributed to the increased symptoms that I now have.

I have chosen another primary care physician. Although I hate to subject any doctor to my current problems and fears, I know that is best. I am sorry to be leaving in this way, and up to this experience have felt good about the medical counsel your office has given. This is a long and detailed letter and I hope an instructive letter, so that no other woman in your practice will experience such a terrifying and horrible experience that has such long lasting medical ramifications.

Sincerely,

Summary

It is worthwhile to note that last week's local paper announced the "retirement" of my surgeon. He's now behind a desk as a VP at our local hospital. So he won't hold a knife again— or ruin any more women. My physician friends and family members have assured me that I did a great service by writing letters to the HMO. The HMO did a full review, and brought in outside doctors to review my case, which I suspect may be why my surgeon is no longer practicing. Thank goodness for that, but how many others are out there just like him?

It has been almost a year and a half since my hysterectomy, and this is what the doctors are now saying. Two colorectal specialists have diagnosed a large rectocele. The last colorectal surgeon was able to pinpoint the location: a low perineal rectocele. However, both surgeons stated that due to trauma in the area, repair is not recommended. They also informed me that rectoceles are a gynecological problem. So, I have seen two gynecologists and one urogynecologist. The two gynecologists do not "see" the rectocele. The urogynecologist can see a small rectocele on the defogram, but not through the vagina, and notes that I exhibit some rectal prolapse. One urologist and the urogynecologist both note that I have a cystocele.

Although my surgeon said in his notes at both my six week and 4 1/2 month checkups after surgery that my vagina was of "normal" length, a urolgynecologist measured my vagina at a year after surgery and found that it was 6.5 cm to apex (normal vagina length is 10–12 cm). I have managed to "stretch" one side to accommodate my husband. However, my vagina is very thin, and very scarred, and I have a constant rectal "tug," which becomes painful at times.

I have had to modify my lifestyle significantly in order to maintain some quality of life. Prior to surgery, I used to lift weights, jog, strenuously garden, and hike. Now, I can no longer carry more than 10–15 pounds for more than five minutes without feeling bad in my rectal area. My legs now feel like they are falling off, and my right leg comes out of its socket when I run up hill, or do other types of exercise. I now wear a sacroiliac belt when doing strenuous things to "hold myself together." According to my physical therapist, who is also a pelvic floor specialist, this is very common for women who have pelvic floor problems, and is all interrelated. Physical therapy has done wonders. I faithfully do various pelvic floor exercises to help with the urinary and rectal problems. I also find that yoga is helpful to keep flexible.

I've always been one of those unsufferably positive and happy people—but I find sometimes I wonder that if these things are never resolved and the bad episodes continue to be prolonged, if I will want to continue living like this. I'm hoping that with the passage of time and continued physical therapy the bad episodes will decrease. My life now is very different than it was before surgery, as I am afraid of hurting things more. Since I am aware that further surgery would not be advisable, I must be vigilantly careful in whatever I do.

My suggestion to anyone reading this, who is contemplating hysterectomy for pelvic floor problems, would be to find a physical therapist who specializes in pelvic floor problems, and work with them for at least a year before deciding on surgery. Only regard surgery as a last resort, after nothing else works. I had seen a therapist for only six weeks before going to a gynecologist for an opinion, and that was not enough time for the exercises to work. When choosing a gynecologist for advice, seek counsel from a urogynecologist who specialize in pelvic floor problems. Surgery does not provide a "quick fix" for these things. You will have to work twice as hard post-surgery, after the pelvic supports have been compromised, to regain former levels of strength, and there is no guarantee that you ever will regain that strength, as I have discovered.

I hope this book helps give women the information they need to make wise decisions regarding hysterectomies. I wish I could have read it before making my decision!

—"Falling Out" - Washington USA

Writer's Profile

ርሄርሄርሄርሄርሄርሄርሄርሄርሄርሄ ❦ ฆฆฆฆฆฆฆฆฆฆฆ

Authored by:	T
Age:	46
From:	Denver, Colorado USA
Hysterectomy:	1999
Age at surgery	42
Ovary removed	No
Age at surgery	N/A
Reason for surgery/surgeries:	Prolapsed uterus
Hormone replacement history:	None
Other medications:	None

I had three medical opinions—all the same. My diagnosis was prolapsed (fallen) uterus, which was threatening to create a cystocele and rectocele (fallen bladder and bowel). I had my surgery three weeks after my first symptoms and diagnosis, and I think that was in my favor for the good surgical results.

Monday, April 12, 1999 I had a total vaginal hysterectomy for prolapse. I checked into the hospital at 6:30 AM for 8:30 AM surgery. Last thing I remember is anesthesiologist putting the oxygen mask on me, then I was in recovery and headed for my private room. The doctor was expecting to repair my pelvic floor in a 2 1/2 hour surgery, but when he removed the uterus, the cystocele and rectocele corrected themselves (as he suspected they would). Therefore, no pelvic floor repair was needed. He was done in 45 minutes. I had no external stitches, and my ovaries looked great so I got to keep them. While I was in recovery, they removed the catheter.

I had some postoperative aches and pains, but I didn't even need a morphine pain pump. The doctor said the pain that occurred with very breath (my ribs hurt) was from the position I was in during surgery. They gave me a little breathing machine to exercise my lungs and keep pneumonia away. When I felt nausea coming on, I asked for medication from the nurses right away, so I didn't have any actual hurling. On my first attempt at peeing, I must have sat there for 30 minutes dangling my hand in water, etc., etc. and finally got a little tinkle (there must be a song I could have sung!). The nurse was not impressed with my little tinkle and came back with a catheter . . . she had a five gallon bucket by the time she was done (okay, maybe I'm exaggerating, but it certainly felt like that much relief!). After that I was able to go on my own. I decided I would take a lap around the nurse station every time I got up to pee. My gas pains were awful and I was bloated up like a balloon.

Tuesday morning: I got to have a normal breakfast. I had everybody and their dog come to check on me. I didn't remember everything they said (instructions) . . . only hoped I was doing everything right. I got two prescriptions: Motrin for swelling and Percoset for pain, and took them religiously. The car ride home seemed way too bumpy (45 minutes). I used a soft pillow between me and the seat belt. Anyway, I made it home and started resting . . . I looked six months pregnant! I parked my butt on the couch and napped whenever the mood hit me. Sitting upright was uncomfortable and I was still awaiting a gold star for my poop card. The home nurse came out to check on me and (what else?) take more blood! I was told to take triple doses of iron every day to boost my red cell count. All in all, I was doing pretty well.

Day 15 Postoperative: I tried driving . . . still tender for me on the bumps. I started thinking I reached a plateau healing-wise . . . and was sort of bummed about that. I was religious about taking the pain meds, iron tabs, and stool softeners. I have wrote them down to keep it all-straight.

Day 16: I started the day with vomiting, fever, chills, and diarrhea . . . even my constipation moved (that was very painful!). I called the doctor's office and nurse sent me to local clinic. When I arrived, my blood pressure was 88/58 and falling. Suddenly, I had five people working on me! My blood test showed I could back off on the iron tabs to one per day and my white cell count looked good. The urine test came back fine. I had an abdominal x-ray to check for bowel blockage and also to make sure my liver hadn't shut down. I was shivering uncontrollably. . . the exam table was shaking! They kept me for a couple of hours, and pumped two liters fluid into me to combat dehydration, then sent me home.

Day 17: I was feeling a little better, but still had the fever/ chills routine.

Day 18: I was totally exhausted. I had gone to bed at 9 PM, hubby finally pried me out of bed at 11:30 AM. Then I only went from bed to couch for more sleep; more fever/chills. We figured it was lingering flu-stuff from Wednesday. In middle of night, I got up for the bathroom and felt a gush . . . it was dark brownish blood. Kind of scary . . . I had not had any bleeding since about five days postoperative. I resolved to call the doctor in the morning. Why does this stuff always happen on the weekend?

Day 19: I got up, but was very tired . . . sometimes during the night this week I woke up in a pool of sweat, I was so hot. I had no energy or interest in anything. I was still having the fever/chills routine, and also puffiness in my abdomen. The profile of my abdomen had changed, right above my pubic hair and where my uterus had been, it was bulging. My entire abdomen area was very tender; I was nearly doubled over in pain when I walked. Saturday evening, I called the advice nurse at our HMO and she said, "Go to the ER." I STILL balked at the idea (it was an hour drive for us and our kids were young) . . . . She said, "I would not be sending you if I didn't think it was an emergency." She used the words "blood clot," "CT scan," and some other stuff I don't remember. We arrived at the hospital about 8 PM. I asked for the gynecologist on call (ack, I didn't want a pelvic exam!). The gynecologist on call was very good . . . he said maybe it is your appendix or something not related to surgery and they would approach a diagnosis with their eyes wide open. They started with a CT scan, which took about 15 minutes and showed a hematoma (blood pooling) the size of a tennis ball right where old uterus used to be. Then, I received a very gentle pelvic exam, as the doctor wanted to confirm what it looked like in there before the upcoming surgery. By midnight Saturday night, I was put on oxygen. The doctors started me on IV antibiotics, saying they had to get a handle on the septic (infection) situation before they could do any surgery, and they planned for Sunday noon surgery. I also got a morphine pain pump to help me with the misery I was already in.

Surgery involved going into vagina, making an opening at the top in already healed-together tissue, draining all the old blood and leaving the opening for later self-healing. The whole thing would only take 15 minutes. I was too miserable to worry about the surgery . . . had lots of trouble with IV's (had three different ones in my hospital stay of three nights, blew out two different veins . . . ugh!).

Postoperatively, I felt less foggy than I did after my hysterectomy and had a big feeling of relief (pressure-wise) in my abdomen. I was pretty sick and weak from the whole septic episode though. I stayed in the hospital and continued IV antibiotics until Tuesday afternoon. After a few days of IV antibiotics, I got a "tin" taste in my mouth . . . everything (even the water and air) tasted tinny . . . made for zero interest in food. Anyway, I finally went home, but I had to go for weekly checkups until further notice. I got to do sitz baths and start at the beginning on pain medications, resting, etc. I was verrrrrrry tired. This complication extended my medical leave from work. The whole thing was really scary for me . . . I had started this whole process as a quick elective surgery and suddenly I seemed to literally be in a "do or die" situation.[4]

Post recovery comments. Things I learned: Don't blow off a fever thinking it's just hot flashes . . . I had a constant temperature! My surgeon's nurse says that in the future, they will send all postoperative patients to emergency room (not the local clinic) for problems. Since the hospital was an hour drive, I was hesitant to go if I was just going to get fluids and sent home again. Hematoma is rare (they thought mine was also infected) and it can develop into a blood clot, which can be life threatening.

My doctor said they don't really know what causes or prevents hematomas and blood clots, so they can't foresee them, and that they were really caught off-guard by mine. My personal opinion is that I should have been walking more post-op (I was kind of a couch slug), but I'm not going to spend any time beating myself up over it. I would guess that the hematoma started growing very soon after surgery.

At three months post-op, I did not have any regrets having had a hysterectomy. We were done building our family, so that part of the decision was not an issue for us. The future of my health (uterus having fallen) was only going to become increasingly more uncomfortable with constipation, bladder infections, blood loss leading up to anemia, etc., with the same final result! I probably would have still ended up with the hysterectomy, so, I am glad I did it before suffering for any more months or years than necessary.

Today, closing in on four years post-op, I don't seem to have any negative effects of the surgery. I made the best decision I could with the information I had a the time. I DO think it is imperative that women research their symptoms and available options, as well as get two or three medical opinions, so they are well armed before making any decisions on their treatment. I hope that more medical studies, advances in treatment, and support groups will become available in order to make the choices in women's health care much easier in the future. Knowledge is power.

—T - Denver, Colorado USA

Writer's Profile

ఆఆఆఆఆఆఆఆఆఆఆ 🍒 ಬಬಬಬಬಬಬಬಬಬ

Authored by: Sheila Leary
Age: 48
From: Houston, Texas USA

Hysterectomy: 1999
Age at surgery   44

Ovary removed   No
Age at surgery   N/A

Reason for
    surgery/surgeries: Fibroid tumors

Hormone replacement
    history: 2002 to present
                       Cenestin® (conjugated estrogens)

Other medications: Zoloft® and trazodone

I've always struggled with PMS. But, in my early 40s, I was struggling with both PMS and the physical symptoms that eventually led to my hysterectomy. The year before my hysterectomy, I struggled with rather vague and intermittent symptoms. Sometimes my back would hurt, sometimes my muscles would ache, and sometimes my digestive tract didn't feel quite right. I visited an orthopedist, a gastroenterologist, a physical therapist, and finally my gynecologist.

My gynecologist seemed very concerned about my pain. At the time, I noticed that I was gaining a lot of weight. Sometimes I would look in the mirror, and I looked like I was 6-7 months pregnant. At least three times, my left leg froze up on me. I would be either standing or walking, and I couldn't move for a few minutes. I just figured that my weight gain was pressing on a nerve. However, even with my weight gain, my heaviest weight was 128 pounds. Over the next six months, I had both an internal ultrasound and a laparoscopy.

I can't remember the findings from my ultrasound, but the laparoscopy findings stated:

> Very soft, globular, boggy, eight week size uterus consistent with adenomyosis with a small 2 cm left anterior fundal intramural fibroid. There was a thickening of the round ligaments bilaterally. The ovaries appeared normal. There was a small adhesion from the left round ligament to the anterior abdominal wall which was lysed (destroyed). Gallbladder and appendix were normal.

Apparently, it was this report and whatever showed up on my ultrasound that prompted my gynecologist to recommend a hysterectomy. I never felt like my doctor was rushing to recommend a hysterectomy. At my first visit, I remember her telling me to try to wait six months to see if the pain improves before considering the option of a hysterectomy. Throughout that six months, my pelvic area continued to pound, my back hurt, and I was totally fatigued all the time. The pain in my pelvic area was the worst. I would just grab myself there, lie down, curl up in a ball, and pray the pain would go away. It kept getting worse. When the gynecologist conducted a laparoscopy and told me I had fibroid tumors, I was happy to put a name to my pain. Based on what he saw the consensus was that I needed an abdominal hysterectomy, because the fibroid tumors were either too big or too many.

I sought out a second opinion from my mother's gynecologist. He concurred that I should have an abdominal hysterectomy, especially after I showed him the four very vivid 5 x 7 color pictures of my fibroids from the laparoscopy. I didn't really care. I had already experienced three caesarean sections, so I was up to it again. ANYTHING to get rid of the pain!

So, two months after the laparoscopy and at the age of 44, I checked into the hospital ready to have my uterus removed. My ovaries were to be left in place. I don't remember anything ever being said about my cervix, and I am assuming it is gone, but I am not sure.

I woke up from surgery with my mother standing at the foot of my bed. The first thing she said was, "Do you know what happened? I told you to use my gynecologist!" Great thing to wake up to! She proceeded to tell me that my gynecologist had cut my bladder during surgery, while attempting to cut through the C-section scar adhesions that surrounded my uterus. My bladder had to be repaired due to this accidental cut, and that I had a catheter in as a result. I had to keep the catheter in for two weeks after my hysterectomy.

Sixteen years ago, when I was on the operating room table having my third child, my former gynecologist told me that I had accumulated a lot of scar tissue. He spent one full hour trying to remove as much excess scar tissue as he could. Consequently, I have always felt that pelvic scarring (adhesions) might be a problem for me one way or another. Little did I know how much of a problem the adhesions from my C-sections would become.

The surgical pathology report gave the description of my surgery as follows:

The uterus weighs 126 grams and measures 10 x 6.5 x 5 cm. The serosal surface is grossly unremarkable. The cervical mucosa is white, smooth and uniform. The cervical os is flat and patent. The endometrium is tan, uniform, velvety and measures 0.1 cm in thickness. The myometrium is pink, fleshy, and measures 2.5 cm in thickness. There is a single round white myometrial nodule measuring 0.7 cm.

During my six-day hospital stay and the few weeks after I got home, I stayed pretty doped up. Even with medication, I still felt a tug on the left side of my incision. When I went back to the doctor, she said she could take care of it. While in her office, she performed an internal procedure and "burned something." All I knew was that it relieved the tight pain, but I believe that she loosened or broke my internal stitches to relieve the pressure.

I continued to go to the same gynecologist for a year after my hysterectomy, but I felt a definite change in her attitude towards me. I felt no help when I discussed my "after the hysterectomy symptoms." Those symptoms consisted of continued pain on my left side, memory loss,[6] dull aches and pains, spastic colon, and hemorrhoids, just to name a few. However, on the positive side, the pelvic pain that I used to have subsided.[5] In that respect, I am very glad and confident that I needed the hysterectomy, since the pain had become so excruciating.

The main downfall from my hysterectomy is that I cannot exercise, I cannot reach or bend, and I cannot participate in "normal" life activities due to an incisional hernia on the lower left quadrant of my abdomen. I am positive it was caused by the doctor originally sewing me up too tight and then trying to relieve the pressure by "burning something" two weeks later. The doctor who performed my hysterectomy had a solution for my "side" pain. She said, "if you ever want to exercise, take the anti-inflammatory drug (Symax) then take Vicodin to control your pain afterward." (That didn't sound like a feasible solution to me, especially since she created the problem to begin with.) Yes, I was mad, and at this point, I was mad I had used her for my gynecologist!

I love my mother a lot, and I usually always respect her opinions, but there was something about going to "your mother's gynecologist" that bothered me. However, one year after my hysterectomy I made the switch and I am glad I did. Both my new gynecologist and a general surgeon recommended surgery to fix my hernia, but after all I had already gone through surgically, I am petrified to have surgery again. My hernia pain comes if I swim, run, try to clean windows, and if I try to sit on the floor to wrap presents. Sometimes my hernia pain even comes for no apparent reason. I am beginning to adjust my lifestyle to cope with the fact that there are a lot of simple activities that I can no longer do.

Three years after my hysterectomy, I still have the hernia pain along with other bothersome symptoms including short-term memory loss. My gynecologist put me on Cenestin, and I really do feel better. I feel like my mind is sharper, and I don't have as many aches and pains. Looking back, I think I needed hormone therapy immediately after my hysterectomy, but it took me three years to reach that point with my health care providers. However, there is not much I can do about my hernia pain other than to remain "inactive" or run the risk of needing surgery again.

The quality of my life has changed since my hysterectomy. I know I am limited in my activities. I know I may have to succumb to yet another abdominal surgery for my hernias. Additionally, I am fearful about what the "new" abdominal scarring could cause, such as, bloating, distension, intestinal problems, bladder problems, more adhesion removal surgery, and/or more pelvic pain.

With all this being said, I really do believe that all things happen for a reason. Maybe, just maybe, one of the reasons is for me to share my experience with other women who may be contemplating one of the biggest decisions of their lives.

—Sheila Leary - Houston, Texas USA

Writer's Profile

ೞೞೞೞೞೞೞೞೞೞೞ ❦ ಬಬಬಬಬಬಬಬಬಬಬ

Authored by: Dany
Age: 46
From: Hull, Quebec Canada

Hysterectomy: 2000
Age at surgery   44

Ovary removed   No
Age at surgery   N/A

Reason for
   surgery/surgeries: Fibroids, heavy bleeding, and
                           rectocele

Hormone replacement
   history: None

Other medications: None

My gynecological problems started at about the time I had my first period, when I was 9 1/2 years old. Even though I never had to deal with PMS or painful periods (PMS for me meant light cramps, a slight change in disposition and, at times, a slight headache), I always had to deal with irregular, extremely long, and abundant periods. When I was only 17 years old, I remember bleeding so heavily that I would need the largest bath towels to contain the flow. Very early on, I was put on birth control pills to try to regulate my periods. It worked! Therefore, from the age of 21 until I started having children at the age of 34, and even after my pregnancies, my periods were almost normal.

The problems started again in April of 1997, a week after my father passed away. The bleeding was so heavy, my husband thought I was miscarrying again (I suffered through a miscarriage, after a car accident, when I was 37). I attributed it at the time to the stress of losing my father. When the problems started recurring, I blamed it on a combination of perimenopause and extended nursing. However, whenever I checked into the symptoms or consequences of either, I discovered that this type of irregularity was not consistent with either perimenopause or nursing. Finally, in September of 1998 I headed for my general practitioner's office. The thyroid, blood, and urine tests, as well as the sonogram, all came out negative. The only thing I found out was that my uterus was retro-versed, however, that wasn't the cause of my problems. My general practitioner referred me to my ob-gyn. He studied the test results and found nothing that could explain my problems. He asked me to graph my periods for two or three months. When I returned and the graphs showed almost constant bleeding, he decided to try putting me on progesterone for three months in the hope of forcing my cycle into a regular pattern.

I loved the progesterone: my energy level was higher than it had been in years, and my sex drive was at it's highest ever. However, three days before my periods started, I was struck down by the worst case of PMS I had ever had: abdominal cramps and lower back pains that were so bad I was lying with a "bean" sack on my tummy and another on my back, with no relief. Then, when my period started, the clots were so bad that I ended up in the emergency room.

After succeeding in stopping the flow with yet another hormone, the bleeding started again worse than ever the next day. A hysteroscopy and D&C were performed the next evening revealing that I had fibroids. At that time, I was also presented with my alternatives: 1) do nothing and hope the fibroids would go away at menopause; or 2) total abdominal hysterectomy. The doctor left it up to me, but did warn me that it was unlikely that I would have any relief soon, since at 42 I was at least ten years away from natural menopause.

I elected to do nothing. Every summer, I'd re-evaluate the situation, since heat and humidity seemed to augment the flow and frequency of the bleeding, then it would get better in the winter. During the summer of 2000, while taking a shower, I felt a bulge in the vaginal opening. I was sure it was a cystocele. After a few weeks of procrastinating, I went to my general practitioner, who confirmed I had cystocele and he referred me back to my ob-gyn. My ob-gyn also diagnosed a rectocele and told me that the time had come for a "little" surgery. By then, the fibroid that could not be detected on a transvaginal sonogram two years earlier was palpable. It was about the size of a three month pregnancy, and growing. The next day, I scheduled my hysterectomy for December 14th, 2000.

I found a hysterectomy Website the day before I headed for the ob-gyn's office. That was the best thing I ever did. I recovered very slowly but very steadily from my trip to the operating room. Thanks to the support I received from the Internet hysterectomy support group, I knew that recovery would be long: initial recovery is from six to eight weeks, however, it can take up to one year to fully recover. I also was reminded of the importance of resting as much as possible, and walking (though slowly) to speed up recovery. My recovery was a little slower because of the additional posterior repair. However, I found that I felt better than my old self by the 10th month after surgery. I embarked on a weight-loss program and, thanks to the group's help I have now reached my healthy weight AND my goal weight. I'm now starting the wonderful journey of maintaining a healthy weight for the rest of my life. I feel like I have most of my life back.

Unfortunately, all has not been rosy. Since November 2001, I have been plagued with incontinence problems.[3] I still have no answer and no relief in sight. As if that wasn't enough, as of July 2002, I have been diagnosed with arthritic pain, most likely rheumatic arthritis and am learning to deal with this blow. Thanks to the support I've found on the hysterectomy Website, I have found the information and support I so badly need.

Even though my story is not exactly a positive one, it is not a negative one either. I do feel a lot better than I did before my surgery and am no longer plagued with heavy, unpredictable bleeding. I have also found a whole community on the Web that has helped me through this. The hysterectomy Website really is a wonderful place, and home to many of us. There I have found information and support at a time when I needed it most.

One thing I have learned through all of this is the importance of asking questions: from your doctor, from other health care professionals, and through researching. Recovery from this surgery was not what I expected: it was both harder and easier than expected. The initial pain wasn't as bad as I expected, and I was a whole lot more mobile than I had anticipated. However, around the third week, I started "feeling" the impact of having had major surgery and, from there, it took quite some time to get back to normal. It wasn't until the eighth month post-op that I stopped feeling like I had just had surgery and was able to get my life back. That's why asking others who have been through this is so important.

If anything comes out from my experience, I hope that not only will other women have a more realistic view of hysterectomy recovery, but there will also be more research aimed at ways to prevent others, especially our daughters and granddaughters, from having a hysterectomy in the future.

—Dany - Hull, Quebec Canada

Writer's Profile

Authored by:	Judith S.
Age:	47
From:	Marina Del Rey, California USA
Hysterectomy:	1994
Age at surgery	39
Ovary removed	No
Age at surgery	N/A
Reason for surgery/surgeries:	Fibroid tumors (excessive bleeding, and cramps)
Hormone replacement history:	Estrace® (estradiol)
Other medications:	Celera and trazodone

I had always had horrible cramps and periods—usually heavy flow for several days. Several times when I was a teenager, I went to the hospital thinking that I had appendicitis, only to discover that it was only period related cramps. When I finally DID have appendicitis, I was convinced that it was only a bad period, and delayed going to the hospital until my appendix almost burst. (I believe that I probably had fibroids even then, and that this was a major factor in my difficult periods.)

As I got older, the periods got worse. The flow was heavier and longer, the older I got. By the time I was in my late 30s, I was having two to three weeks of bleeding and one to two weeks off. I was using two super-heavy-duty tampons and a pad every hour or two for at least a week. This put a major dent in my sex life, to say the least. My second husband was very patient, but it still caused problems. When I would consult with an ob-gyn about it, I was told it was "stress related," and that nothing could be done about it. Not even birth control pills helped with the problems.

I finally met a doctor who did not believe that all of this was caused by stress, and she thought that I might have fibroid tumors. She did an ultrasound to confirm the presence of tumors, and she performed a biopsy to ensure that the tumors were not malignant. Confirming that they were not, she suggested a hysterectomy as the solution.

At the time, I was 36 years old. I was just beginning a divorce from my second husband. I had lost my job, and was worried about losing my home. I knew that I was not in any emotional shape to make a decision of this magnitude, and asked if there were any less-permanent options available to me. She suggested that I could have a procedure to remove the fibroids, and recommended the doctor who had trained her for a second opinion.

The second opinion doctor confirmed that I had fibroids both inside and outside of my uterus. He told me that he could perform a procedure (resectoscope myomectomy) to remove the fibroids from the inside of my uterus relatively painlessly, but warned me that they might grow back, making this potentially a temporary solution. I decided to have the surgery anyway (December 1992), which was indeed relatively painless and the recovery was very quick. I thought he was a miracle-worker! My periods decreased in length and severity, and my cramps were practically nonexistent.

By the beginning of the summer 1994 (a year and a half after the first procedure), the fibroids had grown back. By this time, I was more emotionally stable, and was able to calmly decide that I did not want to have children of my own. I had four stepchildren from my first marriage, and I knew that I could always adopt children if I changed my mind, but at 40, this was unlikely.

I told my surgeon that I was ready to have the hysterectomy. He recommended that we do a partial hysterectomy. According to him, this meant taking only the uterus and leaving the ovaries in tact. This way, I would not need to begin hormone replacement therapy at such a young age, and would have the opportunity to go through menopause naturally, when my body was ready. I also chose to have my uterus removed vaginally, rather than having an incision in my belly (from a laparoscopic hysterectomy). In order to shrink the fibroids to accommodate this, the doctor gave me medication to chemically "force" me into a temporary menopausal state. This occurred over a period of three months during that summer. This was truly the worst part of the surgery, as my short-term memory was completely gone, and the emotional roller coaster was rough.

I had the surgery and went home the same day. I was up around the house within a week, and back to work within two weeks. I even remember going roller-blading during that second week following the surgery. I have had no further problems with menstrual cycles, cramps, fibroids, or any other issues related to the hysterectomy. My sex life improved dramatically, and I no longer had to worry about contraception.

I am now 47, and have just gone into menopause "naturally." I still have not had any problems. My only regret was that I did not have the hysterectomy sooner, but given my emotional state at the time it was first offered as an option, I think I made the right decision. I don't recommend it as a form of birth control, but given the problems that I experienced with the fibroids, it was a lifesaver. While I know it may not be the correct decision for every one, I certainly had an extremely positive experience, and think that the option should be considered.

—Judith S. - Marina Del Rey, California USA

Writer's Profile

Authored by:	Ilene Yamack Kulk
Age:	49
From:	Los Angeles, California USA
Hysterectomy:	2000
Age at surgery	46
Ovary removed	No
Age at surgery	N/A
Reason for surgery/surgeries:	Large fibroid tumor
Hormone replacement history:	None
Other medications:	None

I underwent an abdominal hysterectomy (kept my ovaries) a little over two years ago. My gynecologist had been watching a fibroid tumor grow from the size of a walnut (with the shell on– I thought that was huge at the time) to almost a honeydew melon. It really did not bother me, although I do think I felt it sometimes during intercourse. Then, after losing some weight and not liking the protruding belly caused by the fibroid, I elected to finally have it removed. My doctor explained to me the various options and I decided to have a hysterectomy as well because 1) I didn't want any more fibroids, 2) I would not be having kids (I was already 46 years old), and 3) I liked the idea of not having a period every month. I would be keeping my ovaries so the chances were good that my hormones would keep working until menopause. Sounded okay so far.

My doctor explained that there would be a six-week recovery time. Now this is where I think I tuned out. Previously I had two tubal pregnancies, which were both removed laparoscopicly, which was an outpatient procedure and a few days taking it easy. I figured the hysterectomy would be similar, just a little longer in the hospital and a little longer taking it easy. I even scheduled a photo shoot 3 weeks after my surgery— snapping a few photographs shouldn't be too taxing. Well . . . I was wrong . . . and I did not make that photo shoot.

My surgery went fine. I gave my digital camera to the nurse to take photos of the operation. I wanted to see that big thing that had been growing slowly inside me for so long. Unfortunately, the next day, they discovered I was losing blood pressure. I was bleeding internally, and had to go back to the operating room and be opened up again. The intensive care room was not fun and I remember my mouth being so dry and having to suck water from a piece of foam on a stick. At this point I was not a happy camper. I love my doctor, I think he's the greatest—but I guess this was just one of those things that happens sometimes. Then to make matters worse, my lungs filled with fluid so I had to have therapy for that. So, a few days in the hospital has now turned into a week, and many of those days I was fairly delirious from the pain medication. Additionally, I was sweating a lot—I would wake up at night and have to change my PJs, which was tricky with all the tubes attached to me and the pain and the weakness. I wanted to get out of the hospital, but I was weak and there were so many "chores" to do. I had do a lot of breathing into a plastic contraption to help get the fluid out of my lungs, I had to get a bowel movement—but how to push through the pain?—and I had to walk and I had to eat—nice hospital but lousy food. After a week, I finally satisfied the nurses and went home to my couch.

I'm lucky to have a wonderful husband. He basically went shopping for food or whatever else I needed. I was told to take iron pills because I lost a lot of blood. I was also told to take some form of laxative—Metamucil or something like that. Well, the Metamucil was disgusting and the iron pills made me nauseous 24 hours a day so I wasn't eating. Then the gas pains starting kicking in after a day or so. Oh . . . my . . . god . . .! Really, I just wanted to die. And nothing helped. If I remember correctly, they seemed to kick in during the middle of the night for about 4 or 5 hours. Finally, one night I was desperate and went on the Internet to see if I could find some help there. What I found was a great hysterectomy Website. There were some suggestions for the gas, but nothing I could do right then in the middle of the night. But just reading all the questions and comments on the different forums from and to women at all stages pre and post hysterectomy was amazing. It certainly took my mind off the pain and then the next night I think I finally just pushed the gas through the pain and was able to get some relief. But I was still nauseous, so I called the doctor and he told me to just stop taking the iron pills. I think it still took another week before the nausea began to subside. Meanwhile, I was beginning to look emaciated and I had to force myself to eat (I guess that is not such a bad problem).

It took 5 1/2 weeks before I could go back to work. I started out half days and then the next week full time, but I would lie down occasionally during the day (I'm lucky to work for myself so I could do that). Before that time I felt so vulnerable and weak—even just as a passenger in a car. I tried going to the mall with my husband one day and everyone seemed to be moving by so fast—I just wanted to walk close to the wall for protection. One night I tried going to a restaurant, but then the gas pains came back.

Two years later . . . and I'm fine. My doctor tested me and my hormones are working. I did gain back a few pounds but was happy to shop for new clothes in a size 4 (I was a size 8 or 10 before). That is one positive result (although in the last few months, I've put on a few pounds and things are becoming a bit tight). Another positive is that I love, love, love not having a period and I'm happy not to have a big bulging stomach.

Would I do it again knowing what I know now? I'm not sure. It was a nightmare, but I'm quite happy with the outcome.

—Ilene Yarmark Kulk - Los Angeles, California USA

Writer's Profile

CRCRCRCRCRCRCRCRCRCR   ∞∞∞∞∞∞∞∞∞∞∞

Authored by:	Katelyn Curtin
Age:	Not reported
From:	Fullerton, California USA
Hysterectomy:	1981
Age at surgery	Not reported
Ovary removed	No
Age at surgery	N/A
Reason for surgery/surgeries:	Fibroids, cysts, and heavy bleeding
Hormone replacement history:	1994 to present Premarin®
Other medications:	Agrylin

Seven years before my hysterectomy, during a routine physical examination, my gynecologist diagnosed fibroid tumors. Not only did he recommend a hysterectomy—he was adamant that it be an immediate one. He said I should go directly to the hospital from his office and schedule a hysterectomy for the following Monday. When I asked him how big the tumors were, he said they were the size of a pear and insisted that it be an immediate hysterectomy, stating that they could become cancerous. I said, "I can't go next week. I have a plane flight scheduled for a vacation. I'm going to my cousin's wedding." He said, "Cancel your vacation. This is far more important."

I didn't cancel my vacation and I attended my cousin's wedding. Afterwards, I went for a second opinion. The doctor said I had several small fibroid tumors and I would eventually need a hysterectomy. I asked how large the tumors were. He said the size of small lemons.

I went for a third opinion. This doctor said I didn't need a hysterectomy. When I told him I had heavy bleeding, he said it was entirely up to me how long I wanted to put up with the heavy bleeding. Again, I asked how large the tumors were. He said the tumors were the size of grapes.

I learned that fibroid tumors do not become cancerous and the first doctor had lied to me. I never went back to him.

I went to the second doctor for my annual checkups and after a couple of years, he started to insist I have a hysterectomy. The last two years he was very insistent, and told me at the same time how much he loves to do surgery. He told me this with a smile on his face.

After seven years, the bleeding was heavier and the periods were closer together. When my periods became one to two weeks apart, I decided to have a hysterectomy.

When I went for my pre-operative examination, the doctor recommended I also have my appendix removed while he had my abdomen open. I said, "Okay."

The night before surgery in the hospital, the nurses came in with the consent form giving carte blanche to the doctor, allowing him to remove uterus, appendix, and anything else he saw fit including ovaries and tubes. I balked at this. I didn't like giving someone the power to remove any organ from my body he deemed fit to remove. I only signed for the uterus to be removed, which is what I told the doctor in the first place. I had told him I wanted to keep my ovaries. The medics kept coming into my hospital room all evening insisting that I sign the consent form for my own good, and that the doctor would be mad if I didn't sign it. I held my ground. I went only for the removal of the uterus.

Ordinarily, you don't see your surgeon in the operating room before surgery, but when they wheeled me into surgery, there he was in my face, mad as hell. "You really put me in a hell of a spot!" He said, "What if I open you up, and your ovaries are cancerous. You tied my hands. And why wouldn't you want to avoid the pain of having an appendectomy later on?"

He removed only my uterus as I had insisted. After six weeks of recuperation, I felt better than ever. This was twenty-one years ago. I have not had a problem with my appendix or ovaries, and I'm glad I kept them. They must be there for a reason.

A year ago, I ran into a young woman who had a myomectomy. She just had the fibroid tumor cut out, not the whole uterus. I said I didn't know that was possible, as my doctor never suggested it. She said, "No, doctors don't tell us that we can merely have the fibroid removed. They would rather perform a hysterectomy."

—Katelyn Curtin - Fullerton, California USA

Writer's Profile

ೞೞೞೞೞೞೞೞೞೞೞ ಬಬಬಬಬಬಬಬಬಬ

Authored by: Laura Griffith
Age: 48
From: Huntington Beach, California
                    USA

Hysterectomy: 1999
Age at surgery   44

Ovary removed   No
Age at surgery   N/A

Reason for
    surgery/surgeries: Pain from fibroid tumor

Hormone replacement
    history: None

Other medications: Maxalt® (migraines)

Having a partial hysterectomy at the age of 44 was one of the best decisions I have ever made. My story goes back to when I was 16 years old and suffered miserably every month with severe menstrual cramps. At the age of 27, I was diagnosed with endometriosis, which caused several problems. I had surgery to remove an ovarian cyst, which then prompted the decision to start our family before anything else could go wrong. I gave birth to two beautiful daughters three years apart, and hoped my female problems were over!

Everything went smoothly for twelve years until the pelvic pain became excruciating.[5] I was told I had a large fibroid tumor in my uterus and a hysterectomy was recommended. At first, I was shocked at the suggestion of such a radical procedure, and I began doing my homework to find alternative treatments. I found several other options available, but after evaluating the best possible cure, removing the uterus was the best guarantee. Knowing I had chosen an excellent physician, we decided on laparoscopic surgery to remove only the uterus.

It now has been three years since my surgery, and I can honestly say I feel great! My ovaries are still producing hormones for now, and I no longer live in fear of pelvic pain and bleeding.

—Laura Griffith - Huntington Beach, California USA

Questions to Ask

Questions to ask if you are being offered a hysterectomy only (please note this is not a comprehensive list, and that not all questions will apply to your situation:

1. What procedure and route of removal are you planing to use and why?

2. Are there less invasive alternatives that could address my symptoms? What are they?

3. Is there a possibility of other organs prolapsing or falling down, including my vagina, due to loss of my uterus and its strong supporting ligaments?

4. Are you going to perform a prophylactic colporrhaphy (incision and sewing of vagina) to help prevent vaginal prolapse. If so, are there any potential harmful effects, such as nerve damage leaving my vagina numb?

5. How often does bowel obstruction occur following this surgery?

6. Is there an increased risk of heart disease accompanying the loss of my uterus?

7. Can removal of my uterus lead to high blood pressure?

8. After my uterus is removed, is there any risk that my ovaries may not continue working and I could go into surgical menopause?

9. What percentage of time do you also take the ovaries while performing a hysterectomy?

10. What is the risk of nerve damage in my pelvic region leading to problems with pain in my legs and with walking?

11. What is the risk of bladder incontinence?

12. Is there a risk of developing interstitial cystitis?

13. What is the risk of bowel incontinence?

14. Is there a risk of developing irritable bowel syndrome?

15. Is there a risk of chronic constipation arising from either nerve damage or loss of prostaglandins produced by the uterus?

16. Is there a risk that my sexual response will change?

17. Are you going to leave my cervix in place? If not, why not?

18. Is there any potential for a shortening of my vagina that might make penetration during intercourse difficult, or even impossible, especially if you take my cervix?

19. If you take my cervix, would I experience loss of its mucus that helps fight infections, and provides vaginal lubrication making sexual activity more comfortable?

20. Will you perform ONLY those procedures that are listed on the consent form that I sign?

21. Are heavy, irregular periods normal for some women when they begin entering perimenopause? Are there hormonal therapies available that would help, rather than resorting to surgery?

22. Is there a possibility that my fibroids may shrink when I enter menopause due to decline in my estrogen production?

23. Do you perform myomectomies for removal of fibroids? (Also see next section on myomectomies.)

Additional questions to ask when you are being offered a myomectomy (surgical excision of fibroid tumor only):

1. What are my options?
2. How many myomectomies have you performed?
3. Were the fibroid tumors complicated and/or large?
4. What percentage of the time have you had to convert to a full hysterectomy, because the fibroids were too big, complicated, or too many?

Questions to ask when you are being offered UAE (uterine artery embolization) to reduce the size of the fibroid tumors:

1. What are the chances that this procedure could affect the function of my ovaries?
2. Is there a risk that I will no longer be able to feel the internal uterine contractions that accompany the orgasmic experience?

Questions to ask when you are being offered ablation of the uterine lining to reduce bleeding:

1. Will the cells of my uterus remain viable and healthy, or will they no longer be functional?
2. If the cells inside my uterus stop functioning, what are the long-term consequences to the rest of my body?

Hysterectomy

With

One Ovary Removed

ೞೞೞೞೞೞೞೞೞೞೞ 🍀 ಋಋಋಋಋಋಋಋಋಋಋ

Writer's Profile

ೞೞೞೞೞೞೞೞೞೞೞ   ೲೲೲೲೲೲೲೲೲೲ

Authored by: Anonymous
Age: Not reported
From: Laguna Woods, California USA

Hysterectomy: 1954
Age at surgery   36

1 Ovary removed   1954 (a partial ovary remaining)
Age at surgery   36

Reason for
    surgery/surgeries: Exploratory for bleeding

Hormone replacement
    history: 1980s to present
                    Premarin®

Other medications: Not reported

1949: 31 years old. I bled every two to three weeks. My general practitioner performed a D& C, and found no reason for the excessive bleeding—no change.

1952: 34 years old. Went to a gynecologist who performed another D&C and still found no reason for my bleeding— no change. I was told that abdominal surgery was the only way to reveal the cause.

1954: 36 years old. I began working with a group of all men, and was always afraid of surprise bleeding! I decided to make a date and have the hysterectomy. They found an intramural fibroid tumor in my uterus and a cyst filled with bloody fluid the size of an orange on one ovary—and the other ovary had cysts (they left a piece of that ovary). After surgery my vagina was a long empty tube, which it had never been before.

Facts: At the time, the nurse told me that the team of doctors who worked on me "did in 45 minutes what others took two hours to do."

Facts: The doctor said that there was no fear of blood clots because the wound was not kept open longer than necessary, and I was kept from developing adhesions by "mobilizing" and being told, "Get up and walking right away—you won't tear those stitches!"

Results: I have never felt what people call "the change." I am extremely happy—can swim at any time, no more fear of stained clothes (and after all these years, what a wonderful relief!). I felt there was no longer any reason to fear cancer. I was also told there was no reason for Pap smears.

Sex: I was married at 23 and thought the virginal pain and bleeding would continue forever. My husband could never penetrate as normal (I guess)—after surgery, no pain, but sensual enjoyment, and my husband was evidently happier as he would often laughingly say, "Thank you doctor!"

Psychological Effects: My husband and I discussed children when I had the D&Cs. We felt we had married each other and children were only "incidental." We could adopt when we wished. The morning of my hysterectomy, a doctor came to inquire about my mental acceptance of becoming sterile. I was able to laugh and tell him I felt fine . . . and still do! (I think this is one of the most important things to consider!) In 1971, my husband died from lung cancer at age 52. We never were of the right age, or something, to adopt and he suggested "maybe God doesn't think we would be good parents"—so we just lived happily together forever after.

I am now 85 and continue with a Pollyanna attitude—"God's in his heaven and all's right with the world!"—(well Pippa said that in Robert Browning's poem, *Pippa*). My life is full as I exercise MWF 9 to 10 AM—square dance Mondays 2:00 PM to 5:00 PM and 7:00 PM to 9:30 PM—ballroom dance Wednesdays 5:00 PM to 9:30 PM and Saturdays 7:30 PM to 9:30 PM—go to lots of plays, casinos (love their great buffets), and drink wine and martinis on occasions.

Because I smoked, I have what my doctor calls a sort of asthma/cough/phlegm. Bad habit—wish I could convince the smokers of today just how bad it is!

Hormone Use: I took nothing after surgery from 1954 until about the 1980s when I started taking Premarin. I was told it might keep hair off my face, etc., which I never have had. Truthfully, I can't tell the difference if I take it or don't.

—Anonymous - Laguna Woods, California USA

Writer's Profile

ෞෞෞෞෞෞෞෞෞෞෞ   ಐಐಐಐಐಐಐಐಐಐ

Authored by: Olivia Shaw
Age: 52
From: Philadelphia, Pennsylvania USA

Hysterectomy: 2001
Age at surgery   50

1 Ovary removed 2001
Age at surgery   50

Reason for
   surgery/surgeries: Follicular and corpus luteum
                         cysts (the doctor claimed I only
                         had one ovary—all previous
                         doctors said I had two)

Hormone replacement
   history: 2001 to present
                         Natural soy 17 Keto

Other medications: None

On May 21, 2001, I had the unfortunate experience of being castrated, not because of ignorance on my part, but because of illegal, deceptive practices of the doctor.

When I found out I had fibroids, I found a book written by a doctor in my area who believes in just removing the fibroid and leaving the uterus with a procedure called a myomectomy. However, when I contacted his practice he had since moved out of the area. I made an appointment with his former associate, believing they shared the same philosophies, and thinking that I could have just my fibroid tumor removed without having a complete hysterectomy. Unfortunately, I trusted him and never suspected deceptive, unethical practices.

When I met with the doctor, he did an MRI which confirmed my fibroids and a cyst on my left ovary, with no masses. Without a vaginal ultrasound or CA125 test, he told me, "You may have cancer." I did not feel that I had cancer, so I simply verified with him that he would only biopsy anything he saw that looked suspicious and not remove anything other than fibroids and cysts without my permission. He said that he would.

My only opportunity to sign a consent form was while I was on the gurney, immediately before being wheeled into the operating room. The consent form stated that he would remove a fibroid tumor and an ovarian cyst. The timing for the signing of this form was such that I could not ask for a copy, which would have allowed me to retain documentation of the procedures I was authorizing the doctor to perform on me. I awoke to have my sister tell me that the doctor said my left ovary "looked bad" so, because of my age, he had to remove it. He also told her that he did not see a right ovary during the laparoscopic surgery. He was sure I did not have a right fallopian tube (he was too much of a coward to tell me himself, and he left the hospital without speaking to me).

I am now 50 years old, but prior to the surgery, I was still menstruating and therefore the "follicular and corpus luteum" cysts found on my left ovary were very normal (from the pathologist's report).

The following week, upset and angry, I retrieved my records from his office. The consent form I signed had additional information added to it "after" I signed it. The form listed "hysterectomy, complete removal of ovaries" AFTER the words "fibroid tumor and an ovarian cyst." All of this information was written in by hand. We never discussed his removing my ovary and we never discussed a complete hysterectomy. I wonder how much this was driven by the lucrative multi-billion dollar HRT industry.

I contacted a lawyer who agreed that I had been wronged! He sent me to a doctor who also agreed and said that based on my records, he would not have operated at all, but would have given me hormones to control my heavy bleeding. However, this same doctor said that since the medical records said "multi-cyst," he could not, in a court of law, speak against my surgeon. I remember specifically asking the surgeon "how many" cysts I had and he replied "TWO" but put multi-cysts in my records! Therefore, I had no case to pursue.

I want to warn women against doctors who try to convince them to have everything removed, also warn them against deceptive doctors who do not tell them what they intend to do. I have a bachelor's degree and I communicate well. I did my research, and chose what was best for me, but what defense did I have against someone who lies and falsifies consent forms! My mistake was trusting this doctor.

—Olivia Shaw - Philadelphia, Pennsylvania USA

Writer's Profile

ೞೞೞೞೞೞೞೞೞೞೞ   🍒   ಐಐಐಐಐಐಐಐಐಐ

Written by:	Dawnne Roberts
Age:	49
From:	Winnipeg, Manitoba, Canada
Hysterectomy:	1999
Age at surgery	46
1 Ovary removed	1999
Age at surgery	46

Reason for
    surgery/surgeries: Fibroids

Hormone replacement
    history: 1999 to present
Estraderm® (estradiol patch),
Prometrium® (progesterone),
and testosterone pill

Other medications: Celebrex® (osteoarthritis),
spironolactone (counter
testosterone), and
nitroglycerine (angina)

On July 16th, 1999, at the age of 47, I had a hysterectomy for fibroids. I had spent seven years fighting to keep my uterus, but the fibroids had caused my uterus to grow to the size of a six-month pregnancy, and this was causing problems that I felt I could no longer cope with.

For the seven years I fought off surgery, I was pressured, coerced, lied to, and felt diminished by doctors in their attempts to get me to have the hysterectomy. Friends criticized and then shut me out, because I resisted their advice to have the surgery. I read everything I could find on hysterectomies in the hope that I would find some compelling reason to give in to this pressure. However much of what I read only confirmed my belief that a hysterectomy was not a good choice for a woman, and certainly not for benign fibroid tumors. I tried to find a doctor who did a less radical procedure like a myomectomy, but found no help from the local medical community in this endeavour. I even resorted to treatments with the drug Lupron Depot in an effort to get the tumors to shrink. When problems from the drug developed and I found out about its dangers from the Internet, I had to stop that course of action. Due to the size of my uterus, I endured queries about whether I was pregnant. There was heavy bleeding with my periods and occasional bouts of severe pain. Finally I felt I had no other choice but to have the hysterectomy.

Initially my recovery from the surgery was very good. I felt happy to have the pregnant look gone. My bladder had a larger capacity with the overly large uterus gone, and I could bend over to tie my shoes without having to unzip my pants. I also had more energy.

However, I did develop an irritable bowel after the surgery.[1] It affected me so much that I was unable to leave the house for hours after a meal and eating in restaurants was out of the question, as I found out the hard way on a couple of occasions. It was several very difficult months before I learned that the painful problems I was experiencing with my bowels were due to the drop in estrogen levels resulting from the hysterectomy.

Gradually though, there were other changes. At first I tried to ignore them, telling myself to think positively and everything would be all right. After all, the doctors had told me that I would feel so much better after the hysterectomy, so I figured the problems that were beginning to show were only temporary. However, they were anything but temporary, as time has borne out.

About three months after losing my uterus and one ovary, the latter being taken because of a cyst that was discovered during the course of surgery, I began to have feelings of agitation and restlessness. I became uncharacteristically irritable and easily frustrated, often experiencing fits of rage. Gradually there was a growing mental confusion, what I called at the time "fuzzy thinking," along with short-term memory problems,[6] anxiety, depression,[9] and insomnia.[8] I became excessively shy, extremely fatigued, began to grind my teeth in my sleep and had an extreme sensitivity to cold, as well as experiencing cold and hot flashes. My patience and teaching abilities disappeared along with my gift for writing. Motivation to do anything all but disappeared as well.[7]

My doctor wanted to prescribe antidepressants for many of these problems. However, I remembered from the research I had done prior to the hysterectomy that this is a common mistake doctors make in situations like this. It is really the loss of estrogen that needs to be addressed. Fortunately, I have a doctor who listens to her patients and she gave me the estrogen I wanted. But, it would take experimenting with four different estrogen pills over the course of thirteen months before we found one that helped with many of the problems that the hysterectomy caused. The irritable bowel syndrome, some of the depression, as well as anxiety and irritability have been relieved to some degree with the estrogen pill that I am currently on. At the time, I did not know that no two women produce the necessary hormones in exactly the same amount and time. Doctors often lead you to believe that one pill fits all. Yet, this is not the case. Each one of us is a different recipe of hormones in terms of quantity and timing. I had to find this out from books.

There are some changes brought about by my hysterectomy that I have not been able to find relief from, although, in addition to taking testosterone and progesterone, I continue to try other estrogen pills in the hope of finding something that will return me to my old self. The impact of the hysterectomy on my ability to experience emotions has been truly heartbreaking, as has its effect on my sex drive and energy levels! My memory is also not what it used to be.

My energy levels are so low at times that I am restricted to bed in spite of work that needs my attention and which I enjoy doing. On a recent vacation, fatigue was such a problem that by the time six o'clock in the evening came, I was ready for bed. I was simply too tired so much of the time! As a result, a lot of money was spent on a trip in which very little sight-seeing or visiting with friends was done.

Motivation and drive to do things is greatly diminished. This has resulted in my falling behind in a lot of my work, and not being as dependable as I once was, making me reluctant to take on any new tasks due to the falling energy levels and loss of stamina. This is in sharp contrast to the person I used to be—a person who was known for being dependable, thorough, efficient, organized, and able to accomplish a great deal in a short period of time. Most things now are an effort to get done. Tasks that require memory, especially short-term memory, and concentration are a real struggle.

I no longer feel a sense of connectedness to friends, nor am I able to feel love for those who once meant a great deal to me, and who are part of a relationship spanning a couple of decades or more.[10] It's a terrible experience to not be able to feel love for someone who you know meant the world to you at one time. All that's left is the memory, but none of the experience of the emotions of them having meant so much. I cannot experience intense emotions such as joy, excitement, loss, or sorrow. Instead, emotions are dull and flat, with the one exception of anger, which seems to be more prevalent. There is even an inability to cry anything more than a few tears. I haven't had a good cry since before the surgery! Of all the changes that the hysterectomy has brought, this loss of the ability to feel intense emotions like love, joy, and sorrow has been the most devastating! It is what makes me want to put an end to my life, because I have lost that which is essential to being human—emotions and that sense of connectedness to people that emotions make possible.

My sex drive no longer exists.[2] It has been fading ever so gradually since I returned home from the hospital. At first, orgasms were not as intense as they had been prior to the surgery. Now they don't even happen no matter what I do. I have little sensation in my pelvic region. I can only conclude that the one remaining ovary has failed, and that perhaps there has been nerve damage from the surgery.

I have no sense of my feminine side anymore. I don't understand exactly why this is, but I know I didn't feel this way before my surgery. Now I feel de-sexed, neutered, and dead in terms of sexual identity, or my femininity. I no longer feel like a woman.

I know that these problems are connected to my hysterectomy, because I didn't have any of them before my uterus was removed. Of this I am certain!

Friends disbelieve me when I attribute my troubles to the hysterectomy. They can't understand why I am having such problems when they know many women who are very happy with their hysterectomy. I know that no two women have the same experience of childbirth or of their menstrual period, so perhaps a hysterectomy is similar in its variety of outcomes. All have the commonality of hormones and varying hormone levels. Because most of the people around me can't relate to what I'm going through, I feel very much alone in trying to deal with all the changes that the hysterectomy has caused.

However, I am fortunate to have a very good doctor who continues to help me find a brand of estrogen pill that will work for me. For her I am most grateful. I still have times when I blame myself for having gone ahead with a surgery that I knew was very risky in terms of its outcome. I had done so much research into hysterectomies prior to having one myself, I knew how they often turn out. I wish I had had the inner strength to listen to my own wisdom, rather than allow myself to be pressured into this. But in the end, I felt I had no choice. I feel angry at a large segment of the medical community that does not see the value in a woman's wishes, her overall health, nor the mind body connection.

In the last year, I have developed gallbladder and heart troubles.[11] The gallbladder is a direct effect of the estrogen therapy. I am looking at having to have it removed sometime this year, and I so wanted to avoid the operating room ever again! I had such a good healthy heart before the surgery. Now, I feel I have an irregular heart beat, and was diagnosed with angina this past fall.

If I had known my hysterectomy was going to turn out like this, I never would have had it! I feel I have made a terrible, terrible mistake, one that I will regret for the rest of my life. I feel mutilated, raped, abused, robbed, lied to, angry, and sad. I have so much to cry about as a result of what has been done to me, yet I am unable to have even that release because of the decline in hormones brought about by the hysterectomy, which has affected the part of the brain that deals with emotions. I was told I would feel so much better after my hysterectomy. Well, I don't!

I don't even feel like the real me anymore. That person is lost somewhere and no pill has been able to bring her back. They took a lot more away from me than my uterus and ovary. The doctors also took a big part of me, my humanity, along with my ability to experience life. This has been too high a price to pay.

—Dawnne Roberts - Winnipeg, Manitoba, Canada

Writer's Profile

Authored by:	Millie
Age:	47
From:	Sparrowbush, New York USA
Hysterectomy:	2001
Age at surgery	45
1 Ovary removed	2001
Age at surgery	45
Reason for surgery/surgeries:	My gynecologist stated that her reason for doing TAH/LSO was because I "cried with pain" in her office
Hormone replacement history:	None
Other medications:	Lorazepam (anxiety)

I would love to contribute the story of my living nightmare, so other women hopefully will not have to endure what so TOO many of us are.

In 1985, my then gynecologist did a laparoscopy on me. He found some adhesions and also "minimal" endometriosis. In 1998, he performed another laparoscopy, which still showed adhesions. He also surgically removed a cyst from my left ovary. In his office, he told me the endometriosis was minimal. He never did explain anything to me. He put me on two six-month regimens of Lupron. I felt better.

In December of 2000, he did a hysteroscopy on me, and according to the report, he couldn't do a good exam on me, even with me under general anesthesia. I asked him if he would do another laparoscopy on me, as I felt maybe the endometriosis and adhesions may have worsened. He just stood with his arms folded and said, "I'm NOT cutting you, again." Then he gave me a list of doctors from the local medical center. Imagine my shock when I was told those doctors had been gone from there for a long time.

I went to a gastroenterologist whom I had always thought of very highly. He worked with me to get testing done, as I lived 150 miles away. The gastroenterologist and his male nurse practitioner both recommended a female gynecologist at their clinic, whom they said was "excellent." I went to see her, and I was crying when I was in her office, because I was scared and didn't know what to do. I explained to her I was told that I had minimal endometriosis and adhesions. I asked her to do a laparoscopy on me for that reason, and also because two colonoscopies showed my bowel was fixed due to the adhesions. I had a strange feeling when she said she'd do the "bikini cut." She said if my left ovary was diseased, she'd remove it. I said that was okay, but I told her NOT to remove ANYTHING that wasn't badly diseased. I saw her write on the side of a paper, "possible hysterectomy." A week or so before that, I had to see the nurse practitioner at the gastroenterologist's office. I should have run out that door when he sat back, laughed, and said, " Well, Millie . . . did they YANK your uterus yet?" I just thought he was an ignorant man. Now it SICKENS ME! (How would he like to have me remove his testicles for him, along with most of his penis???) Then he'd see a hysterectomy is not a joke to a woman, either.

On January 29, 2001, I ended up with the TAH/LSO (total abdominal hysterectomy/left fallopian tube and ovary removed). I eventually requested a copy of the surgical report, as well as a copy of the pathology report. On the pathology report, the left ovary and tube were unremarkable (no disease), as was the cervix. The uterus had some small fibroids. No cancer.

When I went back to see my surgeon, I asked her why she removed my cervix, and why did she take so much when there was no bad disease? She said, "We usually do." I had a list of questions for her, and one was, "WHY DID YOU TAKE EVERYTHING? FOR THE MONEY?" but I felt out of line to ask. So I threw the paper in her trash, however, I watched her keep eyeing it. A few days later, the surgeon called me and for OVER 35 minutes she profusely apologized that the surgery did not work. I'm sure she found the list, and I'm GLAD if she did. I had told her I had more abdominal pain and bowel problems, and she laughed and called me her "colicky baby." The morning after that phone call, I was looking at my big wedding album, and it hit home real bad . . . I will never be like that again! I will never enjoy what I did then. Then I slammed the book against the file cabinet out of anger and hate. I nearly ruined my precious wedding album.

Sometime after that, I felt like the adhesions were back and bothering my bowels, so I called the gastroenterologist's office. I was met with, "The doctor has instructed ALL of us here NOT to take ANY calls from you. NOT EVEN IN AN EMERGENCY, until you see our psychiatrist. You have called this OFFICE in

EXCESS, as well as called AFTER HOURS!" I went to him once, and ONE TIME ONLY. I told him that I felt the gynecologist did the hysterectomy for the money. I told him I no longer trust ANY doctors.

I am so upset at what has happened to me. Now I KNOW the consequences of having a hysterectomy, and so many times, I wish to God that I could have just died on that operating room table in 2001. There are so many things she never told me, and I didn't know to ask. She NEVER told me the consequences of a hysterectomy—from the scars—to the fact that you can get bowel obstructions requiring more surgery, which I may be heading for as I write this. She NEVER told me that the other organs can prolapse (fall). She didn't tell me how a hysterectomy increases a woman's chance for heart problems, which killed my mom, and our family has lots of heart disease. She didn't tell me that the hysterectomy would ruin my sex life, my orgasms, and my feelings.[2] So you see, it's like she HAS killed a big part of me. I know it has affected my husband, even though he says it hasn't. I know my fun days are gone. Now, I often wonder what my husband sees in me, or why he stays by me.

Last year, when I had asked my gynecologist if my hormones should be checked, she said, "Could be. Sorry I can't do anything more for you. Find whatever works for you." I went to my family doctor. I was crying and thought he could check me for hormones, and I told him I was having abdominal pain and problems having a bowel movement. I told him I was sure adhesions were back. Then I told him the gynecologist NEVER told me a hysterectomy raises chances for heart disease. He argued with me. I told him the gynecologist KNEW my mom died from a triple bypass, and that heart disease runs in the family.

For me, I am finding that every day it gets harder and harder to cope. Now I experience more pain, especially in pelvic area. I am greatly depressed, more than anyone knows. I start to cry in front of anyone, anywhere. Every time I see a young woman, I cannot tell you how envious I feel. I'm to the point that I even cry in restaurants. So many days and nights, I just get to feeling so low, I wish to just die in my sleep. I'll NEVER be the same.

I reread my surgical report, then study my pathology report, and cry all over again. I read stories on a Website devoted to those who experience adhesions after surgery, and have met some very nice people there. I only pray that I never have to endure the many surgeries that some of those people are having to endure, of which some are a consequence of their hysterectomies. The world NEEDS to know all the many consequences of hysterectomies.

I am so hateful of my gynecologist. That "woman" has taken happiness and trust from me. I am so disillusioned with the doctors that's it's not funny. I am so sure that the doctors had NO PROBLEMS accepting my money or money from the insurance company. THAT WAS NOT IN EXCESS!! I KNOW that gynecologist has shortened my life in more ways than one. I cannot deal with it much longer. I feel like I have been raped. I am so beyond depressed and frightened, that I don't know what to do. I went to a shrink at the local clinic, but he was very indifferent and uncaring, and when I told him what had been done, he said, "That's what they do, even for minimal endometriosis." I am at a complete loss.

Millie – Sparrowbush, New York USA

Writer's Profile

ෆෆෆෆෆෆෆෆෆෆෆ   ෯෯෯෯෯෯෯෯෯෯෯

Authored by:	Janice Vincent
Age:	45
From:	Geneva, Ohio USA
Hysterectomy:	1998
Age at surgery	40
1 Ovary removed	1998
Age at surgery	40

Reason for
   surgery/surgeries: Large fibroid tumor and heavy
                             bleeding

Hormone replacement
   history: 1998 to present
                             Premarin® and progesterone
                             cream

Other medications: Lexapro™ (anti-depressant),
                             Prilosec® (acid reflux), Tricor®
                             (high cholesterol), and Reglan®
                             (stomach)

It started in 1998 for me. I went in for my usual one year Pap test and the doctor noticed that my fibroid tumor had grown quite a bit in the previous year. I had an ultrasound done and she decided that I needed a hysterectomy. Of course, I went along with her and never thought to get a second opinion or question her, because she was the doctor and I figured she knew what was best for me. I had my surgery at the end of May 1998. She had to remove my one ovary because it was so mangled by the fibroid, which had grown to grapefruit size by then. I felt fine for five weeks and then depression hit me.[9] I was put on low dose Premarin pills. I also started using St. John's Wort and pretty soon I felt back to normal. In 2000, I found out that I was already in menopause. I had to go off the hormone pills for a couple of weeks so the doctor could get an accurate hormone test reading. I felt fine during those weeks and asked him if I could stay off of them, but the test came back indicating that I was in menopause and he told me to stay on the pills, so I did.

I did well until 2001, and that's when all hell broke loose. In February, I woke up with shortness of breath, and after spending time in the emergency room and having various tests performed, I was sent home. Later that night, I was finally admitted to the hospital. The doctor's couldn't figure out what was wrong with me, and they thought I might be having an anxiety attack. I knew this wasn't in my head. While in the hospital, I did have my gallbladder out. I knew it was bad because I was told a couple of years earlier that it would eventually have to be removed. I recovered quickly from this surgery, but continued to have shortness of breath. I went to a heart specialist for tests, and then on to a stomach specialist, where I eventually found out that I had severe acid reflux disease. I knew I had it and was already on Prilosec for it, but it had become much worse. After putting a scope down my throat and into my stomach, the doctor found out that my stomach was not emptying the food like it should. So, I was put on Reglan to make it function. In the meantime, while recovering from all of this, I again fell into a deep depression. I kept blaming it on the menopause. I never thought about the hysterectomy causing it, because it had been almost three years since I had had it. I finally called my gynecologist, because I felt it was caused by a hormonal imbalance. He put me on a stronger dose of Premarin, but it didn't help much. I was still so very depressed. After a couple of months of crying all of the time, my family doctor put me on Zoloft and said I was depressed and needed counseling. I couldn't understand why I was so depressed, because I didn't have anything to be depressed about. The only thing that was really bothering me was that I wasn't able to go back to work, which was just part-time at the library. I couldn't make my doctor believe that there was really something wrong with me. I know he just felt it was all in my head, but I knew it wasn't. His not listening depressed me even more. All I wanted to do was stay in bed, and I cried all of the time. I just wanted to die because I was in so much pain from the depression, and for the first time in my life I finally understood why people commit suicide. My life just consisted of going to doctors, staying home, and crying. I wasn't living anymore. I was just existing, and barely doing that. I couldn't take care of my family or my home. I felt useless and totally worthless.

I kept in touch with my old boss and my friends from the library. One day my boss recommended a book that helped start me on the road to recovery. It was all about a natural progesterone cream made from wild yam, and I finally decided to give it a try. I wasn't getting any help from my doctors and figured I didn't have anything to lose. I started applying it twice a day to my body. My doctor also took me off the Zoloft and put me on Celexa. Between the change in medication and adding the progesterone cream, I started feeling better within a couple of weeks. I was far from being back to normal, but I did feel a little bit better.

I finally did go for counseling too. I only went to the psychologist for three or four months, and by then I was much better. She told me I didn't have a clinical depression, and that she believed my depression was caused by my hormones.

I was asked to come back to work as a substitute, and I decided to try it. I didn't work a lot, but when I did it was usually for a week at a time, or just for two or three days when people were on vacation or out sick. I sometimes still felt down when I went into work, but I made it through the four hours that I worked. My story gets better, as the library had an opening for a circulation supervisor. It meant working full-time, however, it included benefits, so I applied for it and my boss hired me back. I started in February 2002, and am still working. I still have down days and I feel like the depression is still under the surface all of the time. I am getting through each day—just one day at a time and I feel much better than I did a year ago. I don't think I'll ever feel 100% normal again, but I am much better. I have days where I go into work and I am depressed. When I'm having one of those days, I stay in the background as much as I can and avoid the public. I'm exhausted at the end of the day. Eight hours is very tiring and I would prefer four hours, but I like the benefits.

My doctor has changed my medication again to something called Lexapro. I have also tried a new progesterone cream, and am now doing quite well. I am very lucky too to have such wonderful co-workers that care about one another. They help keep my spirits up when I'm down. I'm also lucky to have a wonderful husband who had to be both mother and father to our boys last year while I was going through this terrible ordeal. I'm lucky for the support of my three boys who didn't have much of a mother last year, but I've been making it up to them this year. It must not have been easy on all of them watching me just lie around and cry all day, and not move from my bed.

Last year was a very hard year for me, a real nightmare and I wouldn't wish that kind of pain on anyone. I would urge anyone who is told by their doctor they need a hysterectomy to get a second opinion. I didn't because I've always just gone along with what my doctors have said, but don't do what I did. Ask a lot of questions. I wish I would have, I never knew that a hysterectomy could cause so many problems. I wish I would have read *Your Guide to Hysterectomy, Ovary Removal, & Hormone Replacement* before I had my surgery, but it's too late for me. It really isn't all in your head, and don't let any doctor tell you that it is. It is in your hormones.

—Janice Vincent - Geneva, Ohio USA

Writer's Profile

CRCRCRCRCRCRCRCRCRCRCR ՁՋՁՋՁՋՁՋՁՋՁՋՁՋՁՋՁՋՁՋ

Authored by:	Leslie J. Luce
Age:	57
From:	Peoria, Arizona USA
Hysterectomy:	1990
Age at surgery	45
1 Ovary removed	1990
Age at surgery	45
Reason for surgery/surgeries:	Enlarged uterus, heavy bleeding, and possible ovarian cancer (pathology report came back benign—no cancer)
Hormone replacement history:	1990 to 2002
Other medications:	A beta-blocker (high blood pressure) and Xanax® (anxiety)

I was hysterectomized in 1990. All was removed except for my right ovary, which I innocently thought would survive, but ovarian failure became a brutal shock, among all of the other shocks to my system. The doctor convinced me that I had ovarian cancer, knowing I was fighting the assault, this was his control over me, and it worked. He also removed my appendix, and cut a suspicious lump off of my colon.

I was in pretty bad condition after the surgery, and the hospital just about finished me off! One example, I was badly dehydrated, my digestive system was shut down for too long, and the IV needle was in my arm, but the bag had been disconnected and not replaced! That and much more happened! I also ended up with a large ulcerated anal fissure (inflamed opening) by the vaginal wall, which bled profusely, until I finally submitted to surgery again six months later.

No one had informed me that I would be at a higher risk for heart attack and heart disease, which is very genetic in my family. I have familial hyperlipidemia (high lipids), which became worse as a result of the hysterectomy. I developed high blood pressure,[12] and my tachycardia (rapid heart rate) became worse. Being castrated, well, I feel grief and anger over all of it! In my deepest time of grieving, I wrote the poem on the following page that I want to share:

In fear and bitterness I weep,
But I cannot be consoled
A part of me is gone forever,
And I feel that I've grown old.

He said I'd be much better,
When it was done
But after it was over,
My pain had just begun.

In so much pain I suffer, as the days,
The months go by
I can't undo what has been done,
In helplessness I cry.

Soon I must face the knife once more,
Will this nightmare never end?
When there's nothing they can ever do,
To make things right again.

—Leslie J. Luce - Peoria, Arizona USA

Questions to Ask

Questions to ask if removal of one ovary is recommended:

1. What is the risk of the remaining ovary shutting down?
2. What are the long-term consequences to the rest of my body, if my remaining ovary does shut down?

Hysterectomy

With

Two Ovaries Removed

ꞒꞒꞒꞒꞒꞒꞒꞒꞒꞒ   ꞒꞒꞒꞒꞒꞒꞒꞒꞒꞒ

Writer's Profile

ෆෆෆෆෆෆෆෆෆෆෆ   ෩෩෩෩෩෩෩෩෩෩෩

Authored by: Ann Terwilliger
Age: 48
From: Central Florida USA

Hysterectomy: 2001
Age at surgery   45

2 Ovaries removed   2001
Age at surgery   45

Reason for
    surgery/surgeries: Cyst on left ovary, huge
                        fibroids, endometriosis, and
                        adenomyosis

Hormone replacement
    history: 2001 to present
                        Premarin® and progesterone
                        cream

Other medications: Verapamil (high blood
                        pressure)

I was 45 years old at the time of my hysterectomy. I had suffered from terrible cramps with my periods for years . . . and complained about them to my doctor several times. Her usual response was "take Advil" (I should have bought stock in Advil!). As I got older, my periods got heavier . . . and the cramps got worse. My doctor told me it was all a normal part of aging. The pain each month kept getting worse, and lasting longer . . . it got to where it started as cramps several days before my period and then lasted for a week or ten days after my period. My doctor thought I had diverticulitis. She treated me for that . . . then she realized (as I had been trying to point out to her all along) that the pain was totally connected to my menstrual cycle. Finally she sent me for a pelvic ultrasound . . . and you know something is wrong when you have the test at 10:00 in the morning and they call you with the results that same afternoon. It seemed they couldn't even see my uterus for all the massive fibroids . . . so the next test was a CT scan, which also showed a 4 cm cyst on my left ovary . . . not big compared to some, but big enough to be causing me all that pain every month. My doctor sent me to a gynecologist. By then I had started doing some research on the Internet and read about different medications used to help shrink fibroids, and that was what I was hoping the gynecologist would want to try. Her recommendation, however, was to perform a hysterectomy, definitely removing my uterus and possibly my ovaries too, depending on their condition. I had never had children. My husband is a quadriplegic and cannot father children. But at 45 years old, I knew that I wasn't ever going to have them, anyway. Before my surgery, I was scared and worried because I had never been in a hospital overnight for anything (all my other surgeries and procedures had been outpatient stuff), and I was worried about how we were going to manage during my recovery, as it turned out my neighbors and family were wonderful.

Before I continue with this story, let me also add that I had suffered with pain from TMJ (lower jaw pain) and trigeminal neuralgia (facial nerve pain) for about 12 years. I had been through several surgeries and nothing had helped. The last resort in that treatment was being sent to a pain clinic where they tried several different things, finally hitting upon the combination of an anti-depressant and a blood pressure medication, which helped some, but I still dealt with pain on an almost daily basis. In that regard, I'd been to every type of specialist imaginable and basically they had told me there was nothing else they could do for me, and I needed to "learn to live with it."

I had the hysterectomy in January of 2001 (just this week I celebrated my two-year hysterversary). It ended up being a total hysterectomy—uterus, ovaries, gone. It turned out that I had a lot of endometriosis and adenomyosis, and as my gynecological surgeon said—"it was a mess in there—you've been having problems for a long time haven't you?"

Medically speaking, the surgery was the best thing that could have happened to me. I had an uncomplicated recovery with no problems. I've been an exerciser for many years (it helped me get through all that TMJ mess) and at seven weeks after my hysterectomy I went back to my gym. My doctor put me on Premarin and it works well for me. I gained a little weight, but then I lost it again, plus a few extra pounds I needed to lose. Last year I started weight-lifting classes and I'm in better shape than I have been in years. If I had known I would feel this good afterwards, I would have had my hysterectomy many years earlier! And the best part? I realized shortly after my hysterectomy that my TMJ was much, much better. I kept thinking—nah . . . there can't be a connection between that and my hysterectomy! So I waited for a year after my surgery and then I finally said . . . I don't think I need to take my anti-depressant anymore. With my doctor's okay, I weaned myself off of it. We also cut the blood pressure medication in half . . . and my blood pressure is great . . . no problems there. I was so afraid the pain would come back, but it's been another year now, and I'm still feeling good. Life is GREAT—no monthly pain and cramps and heavy bleeding, no jaw pain, no headaches . . . I have felt better in the last two years than I can remember feeling for any time before that! So for me . . . having a hysterectomy was definitely a positive experience and the right choice.

—Ann Terwilliger - Central Florida USA

Writer's Profile

ఴఴఴఴఴఴఴఴఴఴఴ ಬಬಬಬಬಬಬಬಬಬ

Authored by:	Ilene
Age:	47
From:	East Meadow, New York USA
Hysterectomy:	1991
Age at surgery	35
2 Ovaries removed	1991
Age at surgery	35

Reason for
   surgery/surgeries: Endometriosis - internal bleeding

Hormone replacement
   history: 1991 to July 2002
September 2002 to present
Estradiol

Other medications: Lupron Depot® (hormone blocker), Lotrel® (high blood pressure), Bextra® (fibromyalgia), Wellbutrin SR® (anti-depressant), Glucophage XR® (diabetes), and Pravachol® (high cholesterol)

There was no choice. The endometriosis ran rampant through my reproductive tract. The pain intolerable. The bleeding heavy. Hysterectomy. Don't wait too long. In fact, don't wait. So many thoughts ran through my mind. I had heard so many negative things about hysterectomy. Many books advising against it. Warnings of never being the same following the surgery. I was confused. I was in pain. I had no children. I was 29!

This was a difficult decision. My husband and I knew we would be saying good-bye to any chance of having a biological child. We couldn't do it. Lupron Depot became my best friend. Life was better. But the friendship with Lupron soured, and at 35 there was no longer a choice. I had the hysterectomy. While I knew that I was still every much the woman I was prior to the surgery, I couldn't shake the feeling of emptiness. My uterus, ovaries, fallopian tubes, gone. I suddenly felt possessive of my body parts despite their inability to function properly. It was a long recovery—I couldn't get myself back on track. Hot flashes, mood swings, and a general malaise became a way of life. I kept hearing the doctor's remarks, "much internal bleeding," "really no choice," "glad we got there when we did." I tried to use this rationale, and yet it didn't seem to settle into my brain. Somehow, I managed to make it through the first three months.

Then the pain returned. It seemed impossible. The doctor said it was phantom pain . . . funny, seemed real to me. The pain was relentless. I didn't understand. Neither did anyone else. The endometriosis was back. How could that be? The hysterectomy was to have put that to rest—oh yes, for 99% of those who undergo the surgery. I had better odds in winning the lottery, but no, I had to win the right for my endometriosis to return. I cried, and cried, and then cried some more. I honestly don't know why my husband didn't divorce me. Then again, with my hormones having no clue what to do, my body racked with pain, and a heat no fan could cool, he was probably afraid for his life just saying hello to me.

My dream of physical peace, no more injections, was just that—a dream. Lupron Depot and I rekindled our friendship and came to include others such as Premarin, Provera, a brief run in with Fosamax, and a quality relationship with Evista. I tried to make sense of all of this. Endometriosis feeds on estrogen, and yet young hysterectomy/oophorectomy patients need hormone replacement therapy (HRT). Therefore, I took Lupron Depot to shut off my hormones and estrogen replacement to put back what Lupron took away. I could not understand this, yet I followed it then, and still do. However, a year to the day after the hysterectomy, my kidneys failed. There has never been a clear indication whether or not there was a relationship between this and my hysterectomy. Three more surgeries in four days helped repair the damage, but set me up for another six months of recovery.

It has been 9 1/2 years since my hysterectomy. I have never really regained a well sense of being. Osteoporosis, arthritis, high blood pressure medication,[12] all play a role in my body. There are days when I can't put two thoughts together, and there are times when all seems to be working okay. I believe that I have come to accept that there is no way my body can restore all the biochemicals that it naturally produced for me. My hysterectomy did not eliminate the endometriosis. I am still on the Lupron Depot and all the hormone replacement therapy. Is it the best? No. Would I do it differently given the choice? Probably not. However, I would strongly suggest that anyone having a hysterectomy as a "cure" for endometriosis to truly realize that this surgery is not always the answer.

—Ilene - East Meadow, New York USA

Writer's Profile

Authored by:	Theresa
Age:	43
From:	Livonia, Michigan USA
Hysterectomy:	2000
Age at surgery	40
2 Ovaries removed	2000
Age at surgery	40
Reason for surgery/surgeries:	Endometriosis
Hormone replacement history:	2000 to present Sublingual bi-est, progesterone, and testosterone
Other medications:	Not reported

For years, probably since I was about 16 years old, I have had very painful, heavy periods. In 1998, this whole nightmare began when I went to have a tubal ligation. The tubal should have taken 15 minutes, but I was in surgery for over an hour. The doctor said I had severe endometriosis, chocolate cysts, and severe adhesions throughout my reproductive organs. After I went back to see my ob-gyn, he recommended a hysterectomy with removal of both ovaries. I was 39 at that time. I inquired as to alternative treatments but my ob-gyn explained that alternatives will usually only stop the endometriosis temporarily, and because I had 10 to 12 more years before menopause, the endometriosis will keep getting worse. He said that in his experience—the endometriosis always comes back, even after the latest treatments that are now available. I needed time to think about it and was put on birth control pills to combat the endometriosis. This required taking the birth control pills everyday so I wouldn't have a period. However, the pills made me sick. I tried a few different kinds, but they still made me feel ill all the time, so I quit taking them. Then, my periods came back worse than ever, along with the endometriosis pain.

I went to see another ob-gyn for a second opinion. He also recommended a hysterectomy and removal of both ovaries. At that time, my periods were lasting about 15 days out of every month, and were very heavy and painful. I was so sick of the pain and being on my period all the time, I finally agreed to the hysterectomy/oophorectomy (uterus and ovary removal) and scheduled my surgery for May 2000. My doctor told me that I was going to feel so much better. He said that he would put me on the patch after my surgery, and I would do just fine.

I had my surgery at the age of 40, and was put on the patch the day after my surgery. I went home after three days and was fine until about seven days after my surgery. I began having hot flashes about every hour that would be accompanied by a feeling of a million pins and needles picking into my arms, back, face, stomach, and legs. I also started sweating profusely, which was followed by trembling from being wet and cold after the hot flash had subsided. I began to dread the evenings, because I couldn't sleep all night long.[8] I also had this pent up anxious feeling that left me grinding my teeth, and tossing and turning constantly. I began to have heart palpitations and difficulty breathing. I called my doctor and he switched me from the patch to Estratest (estradiol and testosterone) half strength. The addition of testosterone was supposed to help combat the hot flashes and lack of sleep. However, I only got worse, and had not slept more than a few hours a night for about three weeks. I began to experience terrible depression—like I had never experienced before in my life.[9] I lost my appetite and couldn't eat. I called my doctor again, and he increased the Estratest to full strength. It takes a few weeks for the new dosage to kick in, but after a few weeks I did not get any better.

I called my doctor again and he switched me to a higher dosage of Premarin, but that didn't work either. Also, on both Premarin and Estratest, I experienced terrible headaches and stomach aches. The headaches were so bad that I would have to go lay down because nothing helped. Prior to my hysterectomy/ oophorectomy, it was extremely rare that I would ever get a headache. I called my doctor again, and we decided to try a bio-identical compounded estradiol cream, since I was not absorbing the synthetic hormones. However, after rubbing this cream on my skin for months at higher and higher dosages, I still did not get any better.

During this time, I began doing my own research into why I was having so many problems. I thought what was happening to me was rare and I believed I was unique. However, researching the aftermath of hysterectomy/oophorectomy, I discovered that there were many other women who had experienced similar problems. From my research, I was astounded at what I found and that my symptoms were not that uncommon. Furthermore,

I was now at a much higher risk for osteoporosis, heart disease, high cholesterol, high blood pressure, breast cancer . . . the list went on and on. My doctor had never mentioned any of this to me. When I mentioned it to him at my next visit, he said most women do not have these problems—but to me, the fact that I was now at a higher risk was very scary. The younger you are, the higher the risk, because there are many more years that the body is deprived of its natural hormone production. My estradiol level was checked several times and was only in the 20s—a man's level and way too low for a woman. No wonder I was having so many symptoms and still not sleeping properly. I had trouble concentrating, and I felt like I was walking around in a fog. When I went back to work after six weeks, my job began to suffer, because my estrogen levels were so low that my memory,[6] and energy levels were zip.

Through my research, I got in touch with other women who recommended a compounding pharmacy that made sublingual tablets. Many of the women I shared e-mails with reported very good success with the sublinguals, as well as with other forms of compounded bio-identical hormones. I started taking sublingual bi-est, with progesterone and testosterone. Finally, I began absorbing the hormones and my symptoms started to get better. My last blood test showed my estradiol level at 90.

I still don't sleep through the night.[8] I have heart palpitations, and have difficulty breathing. Also, I started having panic attacks—which I never had before. Weight gain is another result of this surgery.[13] I would tell any woman contemplating this surgery to know all the facts before making any decision. Losing your female reproductive organs has far reaching effects on your body, which he medical community is just beginning to understand. I believe that the more the medical community discovers how important the uterus and ovaries are, they will be less likely to take them out. As a result, we will begin to see more and more alternative treatments aimed at preserving these life-giving organs.

Today, I am still on the sublinguals, but haven't found the exact right balance yet. I now believe that it is impossible to balance hormones once you have your ovaries removed. I also have come to accept that I will have to take hormones for the rest of my life. It is very scary to me that I will have to rely on the insurance company to pay for my hormones (they are expensive!). I feel like my life is now in their hands. I did not realize how much my two little ovaries did for my body, as I took them totally for granted out of ignorance. I would tell women to RESEARCH— RESEARCH—RESEARCH before ever having any organ removed. Medical research has discovered that the uterus also emits hormones and plays an important role in DHEA production, as well as in the function of the entire endocrine system.

When removing the uterus or ovaries saves a life due to cancer or a life-threatening illness, I believe it is the right decision. However, when these organs are removed for non-life threatening illnesses, and the younger the woman is, it is hard to predict what effects this will have on her body. And the worst part is that once they are removed, you can never get them back. They and their functions are gone for good! Had I known the price I would pay for this surgery, I would never have done it. I wish I had fully understood the impact of losing my hormone production and having to rely on taking hormones two times per day for the rest of my life.

The cure for endometriosis was not worth the price I had to pay for it.

—Theresa - Livonia, Michigan USA

Writer's Profile

ෆෆෆෆෆෆෆෆෆෆෆ ෩෩෩෩෩෩෩෩෩෩

Authored by:	Anne Hoen
Age:	37
From:	Germantown, Maryland USA
Hysterectomy:	1993
Age at surgery	28
1 Ovary removed	1981
Age at surgery	16
1 Ovary removed	1993
Age at surgery	28

Reason for
   surgery/surgeries: Severe ovarian cysts

Hormone replacement
   history: 1993 to present
Estrogen in an alcohol based
gel, progesterone cream,
DHEA, bovine adrenal extract,
pregnenolone, and
testosterone gel

Other medications: Ambien® (sleep) and Sonata®
(sleep)

I had my first operation at 16, to remove my right ovary and fallopian tube. I had a severe case of pelvic inflammatory disease (PID) and I ended up in the emergency ward of a naval hospital one night. My first ob-gyn exam consisted of entire teams of training doctors parading in and out of my room, peering up the sheet and making comments. After a while, I wanted to start charging admission. Looking back, they probably didn't get many teenage girls in that hospital that provided them with a free show. They originally prepped me for a simple appendectomy, but when they opened my abdomen they saw that both my ovaries were severely infected and one had ruptured. (They wanted to give me a complete hysterectomy and oophorectomy on the spot. Thank God my father vetoed that idea. It would have been even worse to experience at 16 what was to come at age 28.) In the middle of the surgery, I woke up and could hear the doctors talking about me as they operated. "Ewwwww, look at that!" I heard one say, and could actually feel them tugging and rearranging my internal organs. I said, "Hey, stop talking about me!" They looked pretty startled as they rushed to slap the mask back on me. I could only imagine the kinds of conversations these guys have in the operating room on a regular basis. I was in the hospital for a week and don't recall having any problems from this surgery.

Years later, around 23, I started developing corpus luteum cysts on my remaining ovary. This coincided with going into a high stress occupation, which I think had a lot to do with all that and subsequent reproductive system problems. I had a great doctor who looked like William Hurt and who took great pains to keep my ovary intact while "shelling" out the cysts. I tried taking birth control pills to prevent further cyst development, but they always made me sick and sluggish. One and one-half years later, I was back with more cysts. I was working 18 hour days, and could literally feel my ovary twinge when I got into high stress modes. I had relocated and was no longer within a reasonable travel distance from my original doctor, so I went to a new HMO doctor. He never looked very happy to see me, I wasn't one of his new smiling young mothers, I wasn't one of his shiny success stories. In fact, he told me, "If you're planning to have children, you better do it now." The doctor performed a laparoscopy on me and I was surprised when he didn't prescribe antibiotics after the procedure. I knew I would get an infection, because he ended up spending "much more time than anticipated" rummaging around in my system. He did everything but throw garden dirt in there. Sure enough, four days later I was in severe pain and leaving messages at his office. After an extended period of time, he called back and asked if I had vomited. When I said no, he said you can't be that sick then, take aspirin, and go back to bed. It was a holiday weekend and I thought maybe he wanted to get out of the office early. I ended up in the emergency room later where the ER doctor agreed I needed antibiotics and prescribed them. I was fine in a few days. (I later got to see a video of the laparoscopic operation. As I watched my remaining ovary being poked and tortured, I realized that, unlike my last surgeon, this man wasn't taking any precautions about preserving what was left of my dysfunctional reproductive system. He didn't look like he knew what he was doing. When he started to prod at it with what looked like a soldering iron, I watched my ovary sizzle and burn, at which point my curiosity about watching video taped medical procedures quickly abated, and I left.)

Soon after, the real fun started. Around age 25, I started going through what I now know was a perimenopausal state. I started experiencing incredible bouts of insomnia.[8] I didn't want to get hooked on sleeping pills, so I refused to take them. After about three days in a row of three hours sleep each night, I became a zombie. I started having anxiety attacks. I had weight gain,[13] and my moods became edgier. When my monthly cycle came, I would have abnormally heavy cycles and would end up waking up at night rolling around on the floor, it was the only way to handle the pain. Strangely enough, I also developed other odd symptoms like dry eye syndrome and could no longer wear contact lenses. I went to doctor after doctor, and was told the reasons were everything from stress to too much sugar or caffeine (I already knew that I had to eliminate these completely during my monthly cycle due to the increased anxiety attacks I experienced). Did any of them think to check my declining hormone levels? No, and I did know enough back then to ask.

Meanwhile my cyst pain came back, and I knew what that meant. Time to make the rounds again to find a new doctor. This time I wanted the problem solved once and for all. I couldn't keep going through life in pain and having the same surgery every 1 1/2 years. I was 27 at the time, and figured that children weren't in the picture for me, so that decision was never a hard one. Many women are horribly affected by the idea of not being able to have kids, and at least I have felt lucky that it really made no difference to me. Maybe I would feel different if I had been in a relationship with someone who wanted them, but I have not been in that position.

I saw several doctors, but none of them wanted to be responsible for giving a 27 year old woman a hysterectomy. One female doctor agreed, but then backed out, saying she would take out the ovary but leave my uterus in. I would then have to take a combination of prescriptions to force a cycle each month. That sounded like my idea of hell. I went out of the area and back to my original doctor who agreed to do the surgery. I had just turned 28, and the surgery itself went fine. I was roomed next to a woman who had had the same surgery. Even though she was twice my age, we became fast friends and compared notes on things like bowel movements, and hospital meal critiques.

A day or two after the surgery, my William Hurt doctor came by and gave me a big yellow Premarin pill to take. I took it and soon I could swear there were purple spiders crawling on the wall. I had the worst anxiety and felt like an animal caught in a trap willing to gnaw off a body part to escape. He put me on a smaller dosage, and the same stuff happened, only on a smaller scale. Back then there wasn't a whole lot of choice of estrogens to take, so I chopped up the pills in tiny pieces and took them at two hour intervals throughout the day. They tasted just great, kind of like horses urine, which is what they are.

I still had insomnia, and automatically gained ten pounds, which to this day has been nearly impossible to lose. I felt "speeded out" all the time, like my adrenals were on high trying to compensate for the hormonal shock of ovary loss, which later on I found out was probably about right. When I wasn't feeling "revved up," I experienced overwhelming fatigue. The estrogen patch came out about that time, and I used it in conjunction with the Premarin. I could not take full doses of anything and had problems getting an even, consistent absorption rate from any form of estrogen replacement therapy.

I went from doctor to doctor again, trying to fix the fatigue problem. They would just test for blood sugar, say it was normal, shake their heads and look at me like the problem was all in my head. I found a doctor who suggested I use natural estrogen (new concept back then) and ordered a prescription from a compounding (also a new concept) pharmacy. They came in oily capsules and when I took one I went into a complete stupor. I remember standing in a store looking at a greeting card and not noticing until a 1/2 hour later I was still standing in the same spot looking at the same card. I had always had bad reactions to soy based products that way; they make me "spacey" for some reason. I tried Estrace and it had the same effect. Meanwhile over the next couple of years, I felt like an alien from outer space was taking over my body. My hair was thinning, my skin was getting dry and scaly, and my fingernails started painfully growing up off the beds. Sometimes I felt an "itchy scratchy" feeling under the surface of my skin, like my nerves were on fire. A dermatologist told me that up to two years after major surgery, the body might react like this. The problem was that it had been well over two years since the surgery, and my problems were getting worse. In the afternoons at work I got so tired that people were always commenting on how pale I looked. I would get so spaced out,   I couldn't remember the simplest things. I had heart palpitations all the time, and headaches—and still the insomnia.[8] My libido was in the tank—thinking about a bowl of oatmeal was more exciting than thinking about having sex.[2] I felt like an android—no reaction below the waist. I belonged to a dreaded HMO at the time, and none of their doctors knew what to do with me. Their idea seemed to be, "You're young, whatever it is you can get over it, what are you complaining about." My hormone levels showed that my estrogen levels were up, that wasn't the problem. No one knew anything about female reproductive hormone problems, and most still don't. The only books I could find on the market still stated that menopause was all in your head, and the reasons you felt bad was because you could no longer have children. I did find some information on testosterone and found a sympathetic doctor to prescribe some. It helped with the fatigue a little, but caused more headaches and other side effects.

One of the scariest things that started happening on a regular basis starting at about three years after the surgery was cognitive dysfunction (difficulty with thinking, reasoning, and remembering). My memory used to be great, and I was a good speller. I used to be able to visualize things, and I liked to do some creative writing now and again. Now, I couldn't get a whole sentence out of my mouth without dropping the thought half way through.[6] I felt like (and still do) I was developing Alzheimer's. My ability to visualize or even daydream was gone. I couldn't remember how to spell. I'd forget my computer log-on password that I used every day at work, and would sit there sometimes 15 minutes in the morning trying to remember it, hoping no one would ask me any questions about anything, because I couldn't answer them. My reading comprehension and short term memory was shot. I'd have to look at simple items over and over again to make sense of them. I lived in fear I would be put on the spot mentally. I developed a strange sense of panic over the small things in my life, and tossed aside the larger ones. I had a disconnected feeling, like I wasn't in the here and now. I felt I had to get out of the job I was in, because I thought it would only be a matter of time before people would notice all the problems. I'd have to spend eight hours trying to get four hours worth of work done. The hardest part was that I had no one to talk to about what was going on for me, no one could relate at all to what was going through. I have since had to curtail my career path, and have downgraded to a job that pays a lot less than I should be making, but is low on stress and offers security and doesn't ask much from me.

I am now 37, and in the last couple of years some things have changed. I have started taking progesterone, which has helped some with the sleep problems. I have gone through multiple forms of hormone replacement therapy and now use an alcohol based gel, which provides more even absorption. I take some DHEA, bovine adrenal extract, androstenedione, and a whole host of nutritional supplements, all of which help some. I basically have had a hard time replacing the androgen side of things in my system, which I think has been a major part of my problems. I have since been diagnosed with adrenal insufficiency disorder (decreased adrenal gland hormone production), which I think was brought on by the years that my adrenal system was trying to compensate for the ovary and uterine loss. I have developed strange food allergies, carbohydrate intolerance, and blood sugar issues. I still have heart palpitations, and all the cognitive problems mentioned above are still apparent. My body temperature is consistently a degree lower than normal. I cannot tolerate stress well, and have to ration out my energy resources. I have an ever present sense of vertigo, so most of the time when I walk I need to look at the floor or dizziness will take over. Many more symptoms exist. Everyday can bring a new nasty side effect from the biochemical imbalances or from my now overly sensitive system. At times, I have to constantly "monitor" how I feel: do I need more estrogen, testosterone, or progesterone? Is my brain working? Am I tired? Etc. I'm much more hypersensitive and emotional than I used to be. The fatigue is still very persistent. I have seen a million doctors, even some with very high profiles, and so few have any clue about the whole female hormonal puzzle. One even refused to prescribe progesterone since I don't have a uterus, if you can believe that nowadays. The best I hope for is one that will be open to writing prescriptions and trying ideas that I have read about. I quit relying on doctors to know everything (in fact, I think most don't know what they should). I do my own research looking for more pieces to complete the puzzle. My medical problems continue to affect every part of my life. Thank God for the Internet, I don't know where I'd be without it. I've been able to connect with other women who have had similar problems and have discovered invaluable medical information that I have been able to use.

I want to add that the doctor who did my hysterectomy (William Hurt) was a compassionate and competent doctor (unlike many before and since), who in no way do I personally blame for anything that has happened to me along the way. I am different than some stories. I asked for the hysterectomy and at the time was grateful to find someone who would help me out of all the pain I was in.

There are now lots of books on the market about menopause. Women in general are more educated when they walk into a doctor's office, and won't take as much crap. Things are getting better. But, I know we still have a long way to go.

—Anne Hoen - Germantown, Maryland USA

Writer's Profile

ಞಞಞಞಞಞಞಞಞಞಞಞ   ಋಋಋಋಋಋಋಋಋಋಋ

Authored by:	Jane K.
Age:	56
From:	South Bend, Indiana USA
Hysterectomy:	1995
Age at surgery	49
2 Ovaries removed	1995
Age at surgery	49
Reason for surgery/surgeries:	Fibroids - pain and heavy bleeding
Hormone replacement history:	1995 to present Tri-est (oral estradiol, estrone, estriol) and estriol (vaginal), DHEA, and pregnenolone
Other medications:	Ziac® (high blood pressure), Pravachol® (high cholesterol), Atacand HCT® (high blood pressure), Armour® Thyroid, Prilosec® (acid reflux), and aspirin

My hysterectomy was five years ago yesterday. I realize I will need to go through the rest of my life coping with the profound losses that have come as a result of the surgery—a surgery that was blithely recommended by my doctor as a cure to the pain and troublesome bleeding from fibroids. She led me to believe that my condition was life threatening. I now know it was not. No other alternatives were offered to me despite my own research and repeated voicing of my concerns about the potential impact of having my uterus removed. Internet information and the support I have found there from other women these past four years was not available to me then. I am thankful because it has enabled me to cope with the severe physical and emotional aftermath of a brutal surgery. The doctors by and large would have you believe that you have their sympathy, but tell you that you are just having trouble adjusting to a surgery that many women have told them was "the best thing they've ever done." What outrageous and insulting words those are!

My surgery results: I have "moderate" vaginal prolapse, a cystocele, and rectocele. I am incontinent much of the time. Will my problems stay the same or get worse? Will my vagina detach and prolapse completely? All of these scenarios have been given to me by the many doctors I have seen. I don't know. I use medication, exercise, and take care not to lift too much so my situation doesn't get worse.

I have lost my sexuality. Something my doctor swore would not happen "if I took my Premarin." I "had" a strong and appreciative sense of my own sexuality. It has been a profound loss to me and my husband of then eight years to lose that joy and that bond, and have it replaced by anger, tension, a hopefulness that is almost never realized, and a complete loss of confidence and security in my God given sexuality—specifically, an inability to have an orgasm and to have a sense of myself as a woman who desires my mate. Instead my sexuality has been replaced by repeated frustration, and a sense that I am pre-pubescent.

My family has lost a great deal. My three children have lost a confident and physically strong mother. They have lost a more secure financial future. I have cut back on the energy I have spent at work because I am physically less able, and have less emotional energy to spend. Now my energy has been directed to figuring out which doctor, or hormone, I should try next, and how I will pay for them. What is left for me to do? I will continue to try, to take what good I can from life while I am on this earth, and use what energy I have left to warn other women so that the hysterectomy industry cannot continue to thrive at the expense of our well-being.

—Jane K. - South Bend, Indiana USA

Writer's Profile

CBCBCBCBCBCBCBCBCBCB SOSOSOSOSOSOSOSOSOSO

Authored by:	Ellen
Age:	40
From:	Boca Raton, Florida USA

Hysterectomy:	2000
Age at surgery	37

2 Ovaries removed	2000
Age at surgery	37

Reason for
    surgery/surgeries: Excessive bleeding, fibroid,
                            and polycystic ovary syndrome

Hormone replacement
    history: 2000 to present
                            Menest® (estrogen)

Other medications: Tenormin® (beta blocker),
                            atenolol (high blood pressure),
                            mitral valve prolapse), Zocor®
                            (cholesterol), Zoloft® (anti-
                            depressant), Glucophage XR®
                            (diabetes), and metformin
                            (insulin resistance)

I am 2 1/2 years out from my surgery and I feel great! As with many women, my gynecologic problems started as soon as my periods began at age 10 1/2. I never had regular periods, and when I would finally get one, it would last for an eternity. Back in the 1970s, doctors really did not know what to make of my irregular periods, so they just suggested that I go on the pill to regulate them. I would do that for a little bit and then get off of them due to secondary side effects. If I had gone three months without a period, then I would stimulate a cycle using Provera. I hated that routine as much as the pill. Provera caused me to have terrible mood swings, and I bloated up like the Goodyear blimp.

Finally in 1997, at age 34, my doctor performed an ultrasound that revealed I had polycystic ovary syndrome, which is characterized by excess body hair, acne, irregular periods, and weight gain. I kept saying to my doctor that I wanted to remove my ovaries and take hormone replacement—after all my ovaries were not working right anyway. I felt like my ovaries were poisoning me. I am childless by choice, so fertility was not an issue for me. The doctor just said that I was too young, blah, blah, blah.

At the end of 1999, I started getting extremely long (several weeks) and heavy periods which prompted a D&C on March 23, 2000. I had less than one month off from the bleeding, then it started again, and then it gave me a little break. On May 28, 2000, I started what would be my final period. After bleeding for two weeks, I scheduled an appointment with the doctor once again. By this time, I had done some research about hysterectomies on a Website devoted to the subject. The site helped me prepare a list of questions for my doctor. On June 14, 2000, my doctor agreed with me that this was the time for a hysterectomy. Although I knew this was a big operation, I was thrilled, since I knew this would bring an end to my lifelong gynecologic problems.

On July 10, 2000, at age 37, I underwent a total abdominal hysterectomy and BSO (bilateral salpingo-oophorectomy: right and left fallopian tubes and ovaries removed). I was in the hospital for three nights after surgery and had an absolutely stellar recovery. I followed the doctor's orders and took four weeks off of work, and then went in for 4-hour days for two weeks, and then finally full-time six weeks postoperatively. I am a medical transcriptionist, so my job is not overly physical. Sure I was more tired than I thought I would be, and sure I was sore for a little bit, but that was only temporary. Any discomfort I had was worth it for the joy of not having periods anymore. Between the surgery and some other medication, my excess hair problem associated with polycystic ovary syndrome has greatly improved, and I lost about 25 pounds.

I am on estrogen replacement, Menest 1.25 mg daily. I was very lucky in that the hormones have worked great, so I did not have to experiment with different hormone preparations.

—Ellen - Boca Raton, Florida USA

Writer's Profile

ೞೞೞೞೞೞೞೞೞೞೞ ಜುಜುಜುಜುಜುಜುಜುಜುಜುಜು

Authored by:	Kristina
Age:	49
From:	Cincinnati, Ohio USA
Hysterectomy:	1989
Age at surgery	35
2 Ovaries removed	1989
Age at surgery	35
Reason for surgery/surgeries:	Pelvic inflammatory disease (PID)
Hormone replacement history:	1989 to present Premarin® and Estratest®
Other medications:	Not reported

After reading several books on "natural menopause," I became very frustrated when I realized that these books were not "talking" to me. They were addressing women in perimenopause and experiencing natural menopause. I was so young (35) when I had my uterus, ovaries, cervix and fallopian tubes removed that I never had a chance to experience perimenopause, let alone "natural" menopause. After surgery, I experienced a sudden and violent surgical menopause. Reading these books made me feel very alone and even more desperate to find answers about what type of hormone replacement I should be taking. I am now 48 years old and have been taking 1.25 mg Premarin one day and 1.25 mg Estratest (estradiol and testosterone) the next day, every day, 365 days a year for the past 11 years. It took two years of "experimenting" with different levels of hormones and going through a living hell of ups and downs before we finally settled on this combination. Now, after all this time, I am very concerned about continuing to take these high hormone dosages, but don't know how to stop or taper down to a lower dosage. It frightens me to think that I may experience panic attacks again without the estrogen, or feel like a sexless mule again without the testosterone.

—Kristina - Cincinnati, Ohio USA

Writer's Profile

ೞೞೞೞೞೞೞೞೞೞ ೞೞೞೞೞೞೞೞೞೞ

Authored by:	M. Katherine
Age:	59
From:	Jonesborough, Tennessee USA
Hysterectomy:	2001
Age at surgery	57
2 Ovaries removed	2001
Age at surgery	57
Reason for surgery/surgeries:	Doctor thought there was a chance (?) of ovarian cancer
Hormone replacement history:	1989 to present Tri-est sublingual
Other medications:	Lipitor® (cholesterol), Niaspan® (lipids), and aspirin

I sure wish that two years ago I had the information that I have now, before I was scared into a hysterectomy and ovary removal. I only had fibroid tumors, and of course, now it is too late, because my perfectly normal parts can not be put back into place. I have experienced extreme grief over the loss of my female organs and have felt less of a woman. The major change was in the loss of the uterine function during an orgasm. I am still dealing with that loss and work against having great anger at having that wonderful feeling taken from me. I also now have a very low libido.

Additionally, I have had bladder problems since surgery, and have been seeing a bladder therapist. I never had any problems with my bladder before surgery. I previously had two C-sections (the last one 30 years ago), and this new surgery was straight down my old scar but lengthened into the pubic hair area, making my scar red and raised again. Because I develop keloid scarring on the outside, I fear that I will have problems with adhesions later on.

I feel that, so far, I have been fortunate not to have more problems as I have read there are many other consequences I could have experienced. My big scare is heart disease, prevalent on both sides of my family. Both parents have had bypass surgery twice. Interestingly enough, I took HRT in hopes of preventing heart disease, and all it did was give me fibroids and cause the loss of my female organs. In 2002, a year after my hysterectomy, I had to have four cardiac bypasses. As you can see, little time went by between the hysterectomy and the heart surgery.[11] I asked the cardiologist in August of 2002 why things were okay on the thallium treadmill in August of 2001, and his comment was, "Well, something must have happened to change everything in the past year." Of course, the big question here is what is the "something." I am 59 years old. I firmly believe that the hysterectomy hastened my genetic tendency toward heart disease. However, I do have other factors that were present, such as great anxiety and unhappiness in my personal relationships, mostly family, and blood lipids off the chart, which were unfortunately ignored by my internist. His answer was, "Keep eating a low-fat diet and exercising."

I feel that I am a victim of the health industry, a woman who fell through the cracks. I am working against anger as I know that it will only hurt my health, but it is very difficult at times not to be angry. I don't know what it will take for the medical profession to see and acknowledge the problems with this type of surgery; maybe more books like this one will make a difference. However, I think it will take more awareness on the part of women everywhere, as well as more research directed toward developing a good test for ovarian cancer and other cancers. Thank you for the many women who will read this book—maybe for them, it will not be too late.

—M. Katherine - Jonesborough, Tennessee USA

Writer's Profile

ᘓᘓᘓᘓᘓᘓᘓᘓᘓᘓᘓ   ᘔᘔᘔᘔᘔᘔᘔᘔᘔᘔ

Authored by:	Reneé
Age:	40
From:	Oshkosh, Wisconsin USA
Hysterectomy:	1997
Age at surgery	35
2 Ovaries removed	1997
Age at surgery	35
Reason for surgery/surgeries:	Extreme pain during menstruation
Hormone replacement history:	1997 to 2002 Estrogen patches, progesterone cream, and estradiol pills
Other medications:	None

Two years after my surgery, I read about the symptoms of Post-Hysterectomy Syndrome in *Your Guide to Hysterectomy, Ovary Removal, & Hormone Replacement*. I couldn't believe that everything stated there has happened to me. Most of it occurred a year after my surgery. It amazes me that so many male gynecologists don't even have a clue. Two of the doctors that I was seeing after surgery said that my sudden weight gain of 20 pounds in a few months was due to aging.[13] At the time, I was only 37 years old. I never had a weight problem until they switched my estrogen, yet another time, after my hysterectomy. I finally did find a naturopathic doctor, but it took almost a year to lose the 20 pounds that I put on.

My body chemistry changed a great deal after my hysterectomy. I developed an allergy to dairy and to bread products. After I changed my diet, I felt much better. I also found out that many women who have had a hysterectomy may also end up with thyroid problems that go undetected.

As of January of 2003, I am 40 years old. I still have not been able to find a type of hormonal replacement that works for me. I just found out, however, that my doctor is starting to use the testing for biologically identical hormones. I hope to have the tests done this next week. This is the same doctor that I have had over the years. It is very reassuring to me that he is becoming aware of the new approaches to HRT. Since I still struggle with body aches, weight gain (I eat like a bird), and sleeplessness, I am looking forward to finding the right HRT that will take care of the symptoms I still struggle with on a daily basis.

—Reneé - Oshkosh, Wisconsin USA

Writer's Profile

 CBCBCBCBCBCBCBCBCBCBCB   ൲൲൲൲൲൲൲൲൲൲

Authored by: Kim M.
Age: 39
From: Stafford, Texas USA

Hysterectomy: 1999
Age at surgery   36

2 Ovaries removed   1999
Age at surgery   36

Reason for
  surgery/surgeries: Menorrhagia, uterine prolapse,
                      pelvic pain, and history of cysts

Hormone replacement
  history: 1999 to present
                      May-August 1999 - Climara®
                      patch, August 1999 - tri-est and
                      progesterone creams

Other medications: Duragesic® patch (pain),
                      Darvocet® (pain), Protonix®
                      (acid reflux), and pamine
                      (stomach).

My story begins in 1994 when I developed a cyst on my right ovary. The cyst was the size of a plum. I had a laparoscopy to remove the cyst and "supposedly" the right ovary (more about the supposedly later). Everything was fine for about a year, then I began having problems again—irregular heavy bleeding and extreme pain on the left side.

In 1995, I had a laparotomy to remove a cyst from the left ovary. It was from that day forward that I was never the same. The first thing I dealt with was my wound, which would not heal. I had to see a wound specialist who proceeded to reopen the wound and clean it out. This left me with an open incision for about three months. It did finally heal, however, I think that the hysterectomy surgery has left me with permanent nerve damage in that area.

The bleeding problems continued. It wasn't unusual for me to have to wear a tampon and a pad and still change every hour on the hour. My doctor tried to control the bleeding with Provera and birth control pills, but to no avail. I than had a hysteroscopy and D&C in 1997. Still no help. His answer then was to do nothing and see what happens. I was so miserable that I would go to bed crying every night. I dreaded my period as I couldn't go anywhere or do anything, because I always had to be near a bathroom.

In 1998, I finally went in search of a new doctor. I had another laparoscopy to remove my left ovary and fallopian tube. The left ovary was totally covered in cysts and the fallopian tube was totally blocked. The doctor called it clubbed. It was during this time that we found that I still had a partial right ovary. Either I had "ovarian remnant" syndrome or the first doctor never totally removed the ovary. Funny what we find out about our doctors years down the road.

I still couldn't get any relief from the unbearable pain and excessive, excessive bleeding, so the doctor finally decided it was time to do a hysterectomy. My husband and I didn't have to think long about it as we thought that this was my only option. The surgery itself was uneventful. Little did I know what this surgery was to bring.

I knew nothing about hormones and did not understand what was happening to me—hot flashes, mood swings, and my hair falling out. I had no clue at the time that this was all related to my hormones. Then I found a hysterectomy support group on the Internet. I began researching my options and tried talking to my doctor about hormones, but he didn't have a clue. Luckily for me I found a wonderful compounding pharmacist who helped guide me through this process. I am happy to say that four years later I am finally balanced hormonally.

What would have made this so much easier is if I would have known what could happen to me??? My doctor told me that I would feel wonderful after the hysterectomy. "Here, I'll slap this Climara patch on your butt and you will be you again." You know what, that doesn't happen to everybody. Yes, I've done my research now and have learned sooooo much along the way, but looking back I really would've liked to have known the possibilities. Thank goodness for the hysterectomy support group on the Internet!

Now, on to my continuing health problems. While I do not regret my hysterectomy for one moment, the hysterectomy did not fix my problems. I have had three more surgeries since the hysterectomy to try and take my pain away. I have had an incision revision and scar tissue removal. I have had my ilioinguinal (small intestine and groin) nerves cut, and an exploratory laparotomy. I still have abdominal swelling, and unexplained pelvic pain,[5] as well as abdominal pain. I can't eat much and have lost about 20 pounds in the last several months.[13] Eating compounds the swelling. Is this related to the hysterectomy? Does anyone really know?

I have numerous other symptoms that I won't get into. We'll just say that the hysterectomy did not fix me. I have been to countless doctors and have been stuck with so many needles that I'm surprised that I don't have permanent track marks. I have spent countless hours going through any and every test you can imagine. I can't tell you how many hours I have spent in doctors' offices only to walk out in tears.

I am told that I have permanent nerve damage caused by my many surgeries, and there is no cure. The only option I have is to go to a pain management clinic and try to find a combination of medicines that will help me. I am currently on the Duragesic 50 mg patch and Darvocet for breakthrough pain. This regime really did help for the first few months, but it is not helping much now. There will come a point when we can't keep upping the patch strength. Then what am I going to do?

I don't necessarily consider my story a negative one, who can predict what is in store for us? I may have gone through all this even without the hysterectomy. I guess what I'm trying to say is that I think women need to be informed of the possibilities. I have no regrets, but I do wish I would have had a hint about the potential outcomes and not gone into this blindly.

Thank God for the Internet hysterectomy support group, or I don't think I would've made it through this. I gather my strength to make it from other sisters who have gone, or are going, through the same thing. I know that I am not alone in this. I don't wish my problems on anyone, but it helps to know that you are not alone, and that you are not crazy.

I would like to add that pain is an "invisible" illness. People who you meet on the street have no clue what you are going through, and what it took just for you to get out of bed and make it through the day. My boss gives me "the look" every time I have a doctor's appointment, which happens often! He has no clue how much pain I'm in, or why I continue to sit in doctors' offices and still have no diagnosis that could lead to relief from my pain. I often wonder, as I go about my daily life, how many people that I see are going through the same thing that I am.

I would like to dedicate my story to a special doctor. I had been to at least 20 doctors through all this, but there was one doctor who did not slam the door in my face. He actually believed my pain! Even after trying two surgeries to fix me, he was still there. Even though this was not his chosen specialty, he still continued to look for answers. He ran numerous tests, referred me to specialists, and continued to "look outside the box" for answers. I still remember the first day I walked into his office and told him that once he started with me he was going to be sorry, and that I was beyond help. He held my hand and said that he would do whatever he could to try and help me. He has kept his word. He was and is always concerned. He has noticed when I've lost weight, he notices when I am in pain, and he notices when I am having a good day. Even though I am still in pain, I feel that he is the only reason that I am able to get out of bed and maintain some sort of a life. It was his dedication and perseverance that has gotten me to where I am now. It does mean a lot to have a doctor listen to you and believe your pain, and to know that the doctor really cares. So dear doctor, with tears in my eyes, I cannot thank you enough. As I've told you before, don't ever change as you single-handedly restored my faith in the medical profession.

—Kim M. - Stafford, Texas USA

Writer's Profile

ೞೞೞೞೞೞೞೞೞೞೞ ೞೞೞೞೞೞೞೞೞೞ

Authored by:	Jean Walker
Age:	49
From:	Waldorf, Maryland USA
Hysterectomy:	1999
Age at surgery	45
2 Ovaries removed	1999
Age at surgery	45
Reason for surgery/surgeries:	Rapidly growing ovarian cyst, with the possibility of a malignancy (cancer)
Hormone replacement history:	1999 to present Previously tried Premarin®, after three months patch, Climara®, Estraderm®, and progesterone cream. Currently using two Esclim™ patches, sublingual bi-est and testosterone
Other medications:	Paxil® (anti-depressant/OCD) and Armour® Thyroid

I had a complete hysterectomy on April 14, 1999.   It has been almost four years now, and the suffering I have had since could only be compared to a "time in hell."   My biggest post-operative menopause symptom has been depression.[9] It came fast and furious about three weeks after my surgery. I was already on the antidepressant, Paxil, at the time. It was working well my for obsessive compulsive disorder (OCD) prior to surgery. After several tries of other antidepressants, Premarin, estradiol patches, and compounded tablets, I still have had a roller coaster ride of depression and return of my OCD. However, recently I found out that the antidepressants will not work if your estrogen is not balanced to begin with.

If only I had known what I know now, I would have asked to spare my ovaries, if it would have been possible. I had a large cyst that had really grown fast, so there was a possibility of a malignancy. I felt fine before this happened. The only change was my periods were getting heavier, with clotting, and I was spotting a brown discharge between periods.

When I went to the doctor who did the surgery (he was the second opinion), we only talked about ten minutes about what would been done if the cyst was malignant, we never discussed what would be done if it was benign. That discussion took place before my surgery, minutes before I was to go into the operating room! The doctor said, "What do you want to do if it is benign?" I didn't know what to say, I was not knowledgeable enough at that time and had no time to think about it or research my options. His reply was, "Well, you are 45 years old, we usually do a complete hysterectomy." Since, I knew no better, I agreed.

Looking back, I feel I made the biggest mistake in my life. If I only knew what I know now, things may be better for me today. This doctor should have gone over the pros and cons of a hysterectomy when I saw him in his office, not five minutes before surgery. Even then, he really didn't tell me the cons of the surgery. I have since read several articles stating that women who are predisposed to depression, or some mental illness, prior to hysterectomy could experience a reappearance of these after the hysterectomy. This is so true, I believe, because of the great hormonal imbalances that occur. This may not happen to other women, but a woman who has had a chemical imbalance at sometime before surgery, may have it again after surgery. Then, it becomes much harder to control. Compounding my problem is that I am also hypothyroid, which doesn't help with trying to control the chemical imbalances. This also should have been taken in consideration by the doctor.

My only wish is that someday, I will be like my old self again. I keep telling my husband, I want the "old me back." I hope and pray that one day my hormones will be balanced to bring me back to happy days.

—Jean Walker - Waldorf, Maryland USA

Writer's Profile

છ છ છ છ છ છ છ છ છ છ છ છ   ଉ ଉ ଉ ଉ ଉ ଉ ଉ ଉ ଉ ଉ ଉ

Authored by: Pamela A. Sager-Rohlman
Age: 51
From: Lewisville, North Carolina USA

Hysterectomy: 2000
Age at surgery   49

2 Ovaries removed   2000
Age at surgery   49

Reason for
    surgery/surgeries: Excessive bleeding - anemia

Hormone replacement
    history: 2000 to present

                     1998 to present natural
                     progesterone cream
                     2000 to 2002 Estratest®
                     2002 to present Estroven®

Other medications: Not reported

One year ago, at age 50, I had a total hysterectomy. I was didelphic (double uterus, cervix, vaginas, only two ovaries) and was having consistent problems. Since my surgery, I have been on hormone replacement therapy (Premarin) and my hair is falling out (no genetic history), my legs twitch (small muscles), sex is not particularly interesting (just more work),[2] and I am gaining weight. I am a former athlete and despite my age I look much younger. Out of all of this, the weight is driving me crazy, because I am VERY conscious of it and refuse to "give in."

Although I was assured by many individuals, both male and female, that I would feel "much better" without my reproductive organs, I do not. The weight gain has settled to an uncomfortable extra nine pounds,[13] my hair loss continues,   the number of daily hot flashes are on the rise, and my libido is nil despite the soy-based natural HRT I am taking. Sexual activity usually results in a urinary tract infection (UTI) or, at the very least, abrasion of the vulva. I am also informed by my chiropractor that I am developing osteoarthritis.

My doctor informed me that he would perform a complete oophorectomy, taking the uteri, both ovaries and the cervix. He went on to tell me, with complete confidence, that I would still enjoy the same level of sexual intensity as before. He cited an example using his wife, who had undergone the same procedure in her early 40s, saying that she had no loss of sensitivity and actually enjoyed intercourse more because of the freedom from the fear of pregnancy among other reasons. I also spoke with a male nurse who is married to a "spayed" female and his commentary with regard to his wife's sexual behavior and enjoyment was equally confident.

In point of fact, I notice a distinct LACK of vaginal sensations with intercourse and no longer experience the intense vaginal orgasms as I had when my cervix was intact. It is, to say the least, very disappointing. It could be correct to say that I would have opted to have not undergone the procedure at all, or, at least I would have looked for alternatives such as the laparoscopic procedure being done in some areas of the United States since 2000. I feel good knowing that ovarian cancer is no longer a threat, however, I liken the taking of the cervix to the (barbaric) custom of total mastectomy when a lumpectomy would suffice.

I feel lied to and regret that I was so eager to follow my doctor's recommendation for surgery, although he truly believed he was helping me. I would happily accept menstruation again if they could put it all back in! My greatest regret is that I did not learn of the procedure done through laparoscopic surgery until shortly after my surgery.

I would only recommend this procedure to someone who was suffering from a very critical condition, not to the average woman who may only have excessive bleeding. That is not said to trivialize that condition, merely to alert all women to exhaust any and all alternatives before resorting to a hysterectomy.

—Pamela A. Sager-Rohlman - Lewisville, North Carolina USA

Writer's Profile

ଔଔଔଔଔଔଔଔଔଔଔଔ   ୨୦୨୦୨୦୨୦୨୦୨୦୨୦୨୦

Authored by:	Amy P.
Age:	39
From:	Boise, Idaho USA
Hysterectomy:	1997
Age at surgery	33
1 Ovaries removed	2001
Age at surgery	37
1 Ovaries removed	2002
Age at surgery	38
Reason for surgery/surgeries:	Endometriosis
Hormone replacement history:	2001 to present Premarin®
Other medications:	Not reported

Letter #1

Help, I am a 39 year old women, who has had three different surgeries, in the removal of my female organs, but since my last surgery, I suffer from extreme menopausal problems. First, I had extreme hot flashes and night sweats, even though I was taking high doses of hormone replacement therapy. Now, I am suffering from continual bacterial, and yeast infections, extreme vaginal and vulva dryness, no sex drive,[2] or very low sexual desire. I had my hormone levels checked, thyroid, etc. They are all within the normal range. Nothing that I do or take seems to clear or alleviate these conditions.

All of this is causing extreme havoc to my marriage. I need to find a doctor that specializes in menopausal related problems. My regular doctor is even stumped. Please help. I'm in desperate need of help.

Letter #2

Hi! I was really glad to finally get a response from someone. I wrote to several of the medical and health sites on the Internet and no one would respond to my peculiar problem, or even send me some information as to where I could find a doctor who specializes in the kind of problems that I am experiencing.

The continual bacterial vaginosis has been ongoing for over six months. I am going broke because of repeated follow-ups and continual lab charges for cultures to see if I still have the infections, which I always do. So, then I have to pay for medications again, and again. I can't remember what it is like not to have to be on medications. My doctor finally referred me to the local university medical center, but I can't even get in there for two months. In the mean time, this is really causing me a lot of unnecessary stress and financial expense, not to mention how this is affecting my marriage. I am really considering ending my

184   HYSTERECTOMY? THE BEST OR WORST...

marriage, because I feel guilt over not being able to meet my husband's needs. It is really bad to look like a woman, and have the thoughts of desire, but have a body that won't cooperate. Yet, even when I do have that little flame spark, I can't anyway, because I am plagued with constant infections.

If my story can be of use in your book and could help someone else in my situation, you have more than my permission, you have my gratitude. I sincerely appreciate your taking the time to reply to my letter. It is more consideration than I have been given thus far, even by the medical profession. Thank you.

—Amy P. - Boise, Idaho USA

Writer's Profile

෴෴෴෴෴෴෴෴෴෴෴   🍒   ෴෴෴෴෴෴෴෴෴෴෴

Authored by:	Nancy H.
Age:	48
From:	Flushing, Michigan USA
Hysterectomy:	2001
Age at surgery	46
2 Ovaries removed	2001
Age at surgery	46
Reason for surgery/surgeries:	Heavy bleeding, numerous fibroids, and enlarged uterus
Hormone replacement history:	2001 to present Prempro™
Other medications:	Xanax® (anxiety attacks)

My medical problems started innocently enough in my early 40s. At the time, I started experiencing many symptoms of early menopause. When I talked to my doctor about this, his answer was to put me on Premarin to see if that made any difference. It did, and I was very happy at that point.

Over the next couple of years, my bleeding started to become more and more irregular. I had days so heavy that I couldn't even leave the house, and my cycle was lasting longer due to spotting before and after my actual period. We moved during this time and I had to see a new doctor. She continued me on the Premarin because it had helped me in the past.

Still my periods became worse and worse. The new doctor decided to run some tests to see what was going on. It was discovered that I had numerous fibroids and an enlarged uterus. We tried several different treatments, each involving different levels and types of HRT. None of these did anything to help my monthly cycle. If anything, each treatment seemed to make matters worse.

I was finally sent to a surgeon and was given two options: 1) A D&C, which he said might or might not help, but could provide some symptom relief for a few years until I went into a more active menopause, at which time the fibroids can shrink. 2) I could have a hysterectomy, which would take care of the fibroid problem completely. He did stress to me how major a surgery this would be. He left the options up to me. I decided that since I had tried all the other options, that I would give the D&C a try, just to make sure I had tried everything possible before having major surgery.

I had the D&C late in December of 2000. I had a very easy time with it. I was even able to go out for dinner that evening. I felt like maybe this could be my solution.

About two weeks later, I started what turned out to be the worst period I had ever had. The D&C had not helped at all. Again, the treatment seemed to just make matter worse. I called my surgeon's office and told them I was ready to go ahead and schedule the hysterectomy. They called three days later with my surgery date, and all my dates for my visits to the surgeon and to the hospital for all my pre-op work. This is when my panic really started to set in. I had never had any type of major surgery, and I realized I was more afraid of just having surgery than I was of the actual hysterectomy recovery.

At this point in my life, having more children wasn't an option I wanted anymore, so that emotion didn't play into my hysterectomy. My daughter was 19 at the time and away at college. My stepdaughter was married and had made us grandparents by the time my hysterectomy was scheduled. My husband and I were actually enjoying the empty nest syndrome. It had been a long time since we had just been a couple.

I frantically searched the Internet for information concerning hysterectomies. I found medical sites which either talked in medical terms that were both confusing and scary, or I found sites which really didn't tell me much of anything. Fortunately, I found a hysterectomy Website about one month before my surgery. I read everything on the site. I asked questions of ladies who had just been through the surgery, and learned many things to do and not to do. By the time I was ready to head off to the hospital, I felt ready.

My doctor was great. He had told me many things and left himself open to answer questions, of which I had many. As I was being put to sleep, he patted my hand and told me he would take good care of me. As I drifted off, I felt safe in his care and his medical knowledge.

I woke up in recovery in more pain than I had anticipated. My doctor found, once he was inside, that I also had tons of endometriosis. I had no symptoms of this, so it was quite a shock for both of us. He had to laser it off most of my lower abdomen. It took several hours to get my pain medications caught up with my level of pain, but the nurses were great and didn't give up until I didn't hurt. I had my pain pump at my hand, and I felt pretty good now.

My doctor stressed the importance of walking afterwards as did all the ladies at on the hysterectomy Internet chat room. I was a walker before my surgery and really wanted to resume it almost immediately. The nurse came into my room at 8:00 the evening of my hysterectomy and asked me if I wanted to try to get up and move around some. My head was screaming "No!" but I knew I should try. With a little help, I was able to sit up, then stand up. I got slightly nauseous, but was given a shot for that and it passed quickly. Not only did I stand that night, I stood up straight and walked down the hall part of the way and then back to my room. I knew I was going to be okay.

My surgery was on Tuesday March 6th, 2001, and I came home from the hospital on Thursday the 8th. I followed every rule given me by the nurses, the doctor's office, and the hysterectomy Website. I rested and took time for myself to heal for the entire next six weeks. When I went back for my final checkup, my doctor wanted to know if he could make me his poster child for hysterectomies. This made me feel good. I knew I had healed well, and I was hopeful I wouldn't have any complications down the road.

Over the entire year following my hysterectomy I continued to listen to my body. If I found something hurt or even caused me discomfort, I'd stop doing it. Carrying luggage at the airport when I was 7 1/2 months post-op caused me to have some pains that stopped me in my tracks. I hadn't had those in a long time, and had to tell my husband that I couldn't lift any more suitcases on the trip. He was great throughout my entire recovery, and I owe him so much for being there completely for me.

At 22 months postoperative, I have no problems with my recovery. I was put on Prempro to help stave off any recurring endometriosis. I am glad I had my hysterectomy, because I feel I have my life back. My days are not spent worrying about when

I'm going to start my period. When a social engagement comes up, I don't immediately have to look at the calendar to see if I'm going to be bleeding too heavily to even be able to attend. I find I don't know where all the bathrooms are at the places we have visited since my hysterectomy. I am a true success story.

—Nancy H. - Flushing, Michigan USA

Writer's Profile

ෆෆෆෆෆෆෆෆෆෆෆ ෩෩෩෩෩෩෩෩෩෩෩

Authored by:	Teresa Masonia
Age:	39
From:	Killen, Alabama USA
Hysterectomy:	1996
Age at surgery	32
2 Ovaries removed	2001
Age at surgery	37
Reason for surgery/surgeries:	Endometriosis
Hormone replacement history:	2001 to present Premarin®
Other medications:	Prozac® (depression)

I am 38 years old. I had a hysterectomy (still had my ovaries) in 1996. After my surgery, I initially felt fine. Then about two years ago I began to hurt from endometriosis. I tolerated the pain as long as I possibly could. So in May of 2001, I had my ovaries removed also. My doctor did not want to take my ovaries, but had no choice due to endometriosis and scar tissue. I felt great right after my surgery, and I thought this was the best thing I could have done.

Two months later, in July 2001, I started a new job and was very excited about it, and for the first time in a long while I thought my life was going to be great. In September, I began to have really bad mood swings, hot flashes, trouble sleeping,[8] gaining weight,[13] fatigue, depression,[9] and had absolutely no libido.[2] At first, I would have just one bad day during the week, then it became two, or three bad days a week. I became very withdrawn, I did not want to be around anyone else. I did not even want to be around myself.

I have taken numerous prescription drugs trying to find one that will eliminate these symptoms, including: Premarin, Estratest, customized prescriptions, and progesterone cream. None of them worked for me. Then I read *Your Guide to Hysterectomy, Ovary Removal, & Hormone Replacement* and realized there were more hormone choices. So, I tried the Climara patch, which left me feeling great the first day I put it on, but very fatigued for the rest of the days. I tried using the Vivelle patches, and they seemed to be doing better than anything else I had tried so far.

I have been exercising regularly, trying to get this weight off and to help with my mood swings, along with taking Prozac. I still feel like I need something different, due to no libido, and the weight gain that I cannot seem to lose.

In April 2003, I have an appointment with a hormone specialist that is 2 1/2 hours from where I live, which is the closest one I could find.

I am confident that there is hope out there. Your book has let me know that other women are having the same problems I am having and they have found help. Along with yours, I have read numerous other books and articles on this subject trying to educate myself. Even though I have learned a lot, I realize I need a specialist to check my blood for hormone levels.

In addition, I have since been to a doctor and was told that most women my age are not getting enough estrogen. I am currently on Premarin 1.25 mg a day and seem to have more energy, but I am still not my old self. Hopefully I will soon get back to myself, because I do feel like a totally different person since my surgery. However, it is a lot better than a year ago. I urge women to check all options before deciding on a final hysterectomy procedure.

Teresa Masonia - Killen, Alabama USA

Writer's Profile

ⳗⳗⳗⳗⳗⳗⳗⳗⳗⳗⳗ   ⳍⳍⳍⳍⳍⳍⳍⳍⳍⳍ

Authored by: Philippa Joyce
Age: 46
From: Amersham, Buckinghamshire
                     UK

Hysterectomy: 1996
Age at surgery   40

2 Ovaries removed   1996
Age at surgery   40

Reason for
    surgery/surgeries: Severe pre-menstrual
                     syndrome (PMS)

Hormone replacement
    history: 1991 to 2001
                     Estradiol only

                     2001 to present
                     Estradiol gel, progesterone and
                     testosterone cream

Other medications: Not reported

I am very ashamed of the fact that I actually requested a hysterectomy for menstrual problems relating to pre-menstrual syndrome and postnatal depression. I did so because the operation had helped a friend of mine with heavy bleeding, and I was at my wits end for a solution to my problems. I had my ovaries removed at the same time—they explained to me the night before the operation that it was better to take them at the same time due to the risk of cancer. I went along with this recommendation and gave my consent without checking with anybody else, which I regret deeply. Now six years later, I realize that my 30-year misery of pre-menstrual problems was most likely caused by my body's lack of progesterone (probably caused by going on birth control pills), and other issues that I had to deal with in my life.

To explain in a little more detail, my doctor had prescribed hormone replacement therapy (estrogen only) in an attempt to help with severe postnatal depression after the birth of my second baby. This appeared to help for a year or two, but after two to three years, my body could not cope with this excess of estrogen and I feel I went into what has been termed as "estrogen dominance." During a very busy period at work, or when a family problem occurred, I found I was unable to deal with the stress, and my immune system was affected, which gave me constant infections. I also have severe energy level swings on a daily basis, going from very high energy one day, to very low the next. I always thought my problems were hormone related and getting rid of my whole reproductive system appeared to be a good solution. The medical justification was to enable me to stay on "estrogen only" treatment, (as there is high likelihood for estrogen to cause cancer of the uterus when it is not combined with progesterone). I have since read that this is a terrible justification for the operation, as no one should be on estrogen only anyway. If only I had researched the operation myself, and understood its consequences before my surgery (I now have the Internet).

I was given just estrogen after the operation, but in too high a dose. It was only after my symptoms started to reappear and after five years of unexplained weight gain that I researched the Internet and found that natural progesterone is needed to balance a much smaller amount of estrogen. In addition to estrogen and progesterone, I now also take tiny amounts of testosterone once a week.

In summary, I wish I had tried more alternatives before embarking on such a major operation.

—Philippa Joyce - Amersham, Buckinghamshire UK

Writer's Profile

ಚ3ಚ3ಚ3ಚ3ಚ3ಚ3ಚ3ಚ3ಚ3ಚ3ಚ3   ಖುಖುಖುಖುಖುಖುಖುಖುಖುಖು

Authored by:	Patricia Zabaldo
Age:	53
From:	Markato, Kansas USA
Hysterectomy:	1988
Age at surgery	38
1 Ovary removed	1988
Age at surgery	38
1 Ovary removed	1995
Age at surgery	45
Reason for surgery/surgeries:	Excessive bleeding
Hormone replacement history:	1995 to present Estradiol
Other medications:	Prozac® (anti-depressant), Ambien® (sleep), and Prilosec® (acid reflux)

I am a 53 year old woman who had a hysterectomy in 1988 when I was 38. I was bleeding everyday throughout the last four years before the surgery. I tried everything to control the bleeding. Birth control pills were the last thing I used, and they did work for about a year. After that year, I started with the uncontrollable bleeding again. Since my hysterectomy, I have felt as if the doctors killed me. I am nothing like I was before the surgery. I am not the thin, beautiful, vibrant, happy-go-lucky, carefree, laughing at life kind of person like I use to be. Now, I sit a home and NEVER want to leave my home, and I have lost all my friends. I had a very active sex drive before the surgery and none afterwards.[2] They took my left ovary and uterus out during the first surgery. The doctors said my right ovary was fine. Yeah right. I never felt the same even with one ovary left.

I almost died when I had my hysterectomy and stayed in the hospital for seven days.[4] Morphine did not work to help with my pain. So, the nurses kept giving me morphine over and over until my blood pressure got so low that they did a code blue on me! The hysterectomy did kill the woman that I once was. I was energetic—now I have chronic fatigue syndrome and fibromyalgia. I was a workaholic—now I can hardly walk to the bathroom without my cane or someone else helping me. I had to go on disability in 1995 due to fibromyalgia and chronic fatigue syndrome. I am hospitalized almost monthly for dehydration, and yet the doctor does not try to cure the symptom, he just covers it up.

About five years after the hysterectomy I went to another doctor and he said my right ovary had to come out. He was an honest doctor at least, and told me that women should never have a partial hysterectomy, because within five years they will have to come back and have the rest of their female organs removed. When I had my right ovary out, it was to be a simple surgery. It turned into a long surgery because the doctor was using a laser and couldn't find my ovary, which by the time of the second surgery had become infected and was black. It had been doing no good in my body, and was just making me sick.

My husband at the time of my hysterectomy is now my boyfriend. He loves sex—I hate it now. My desire for sex was what attracted us to each other in the first place—the more the better. Now, I never feel the urge. I have gone from doctor to doctor since my hysterectomy to beg for the right hormone therapy for my system. I have begged for something to just make me have a sex drive again. No luck. Not one doctor has taken me seriously. I have tried testosterone shots, I've even tried Viagra and still nothing has brought me back to the vibrant, sensual, and sexual woman I use to be.

I feel to this day, if I had to choose between having a period everyday, or living like I live now, I would have NEVER chosen to agree with the doctors and have the surgery done.

I beg every woman out there to do as much research as you can, and try to keep all of your female parts as long as you can, and never listen to the first doctor who says you must have a hysterectomy. It destroyed my life as I once knew it. I wouldn't wish for any other woman to suffer like I have all these years.

—Patricia Zabaldo – Markato, Kansas USA

Writer's Profile

ങങങങങങങങങങ 🐛 ാാാാാാാാാാ

Authored by:	Mary
Age:	52
From:	St. Paul, Minnesota USA
Hysterectomy:	1997
Age at surgery	47
2 Ovaries removed	1997
Age at surgery	47
Reason for surgery/surgeries:	Prolapsed uterus
Hormone replacement history:	1997 to present
Other medications:	Not reported

Around the fall of 1996, I suspected I had a prolapsed uterus and asked my internist for a recommendation for a gynecologist. He suggested a young female gynecologist at the same clinic. I set up an appointment with her and she seemed very nice and caring. I had heard that sometimes hysterectomies were unnecessary, I figured my best protection against that was to have a young woman doctor. I believed that she would be up to date on all the pertinent medical knowledge, and I trusted that another woman would not perform an unnecessary surgery.

At my first appointment she examined me and confirmed that I did have a prolapsed uterus. She told me that there were only two ways to correct it: 1) inserting a pessary or 2) a hysterectomy. She went on to say that a pessary could not be used by a sexually active woman—which left me with only one choice. I was only 47 and not ready to give up that part of my life. My first question to her was whether or not it would affect my sexuality. She assured me it would not.

At my pre-op physical in February of 1997, I asked her again if the surgery would affect me sexually. She laughed and assured me it would not (giving me the distinct impression that it was a stupid question). She did tell me that side effects I might experience were hot flashes and night sweats, which she said would be minimized by estrogen therapy. She said we should discuss hormone replacement therapy and I told her that my internist said I had no choice. With my history of rheumatoid arthritis and long-term use of steroids, he felt it was an absolute must. She agreed and never said anything more about it. She did not give me any information on the risks associated with HRT. Just because I had to have it, did not absolve her of the obligation to explain the risks and benefits associated with HRT. She also said we had to talk about my ovaries and if they should be removed. At my first visit, they had done tests to determine my hormone levels. She told me those tests showed that my ovaries were no longer working (not true). She went on to tell me how deadly ovarian cancer was and that by the time it's discovered, it's usually too late to save a woman's life. I replied, "You said my ovaries aren't working and ovarian cancer is so deadly, why wouldn't you remove them?" She just nodded and said they would remove them . . . like they were relieving me of some terrible burden. I'm embarrassed to say it, but that was the extent of our discussion. I didn't know enough about my own body to ask the right questions, and she wasn't about to volunteer any information to "muddy the waters."

This was a surgery I was anxious to have. I had heard many "happy hysterectomy" stories. For years my arthritis was always worse just before and during my periods and I had a very heavy feeling down into my legs. I had no feelings of sadness, since my children were nearly grown and I didn't want anymore. I was looking forward to a second honeymoon with my husband. I felt I was sliding very smoothly into middle age.

After the surgery, I woke up feeling very agitated and anxious. I couldn't sleep and felt weird. A nurse came in and said that if I wasn't going to sleep, I might as well do some reading, so she gave me two pamphlets—one on menopause and one on hysterectomy. I started reading and really got anxious. Both brochures talked about loss of libido, incontinence, fatigue, hair loss, and lots of other lovely things, which my doctor never mentioned. This made me feel even more anxious, although I was so doped up, I didn't say much at first. When my doctor came to see me the next day, I showed her the pamphlet on hysterectomy (which showed various degrees of hysterectomy) and asked her about my cervix. She looked at me and said, "You don't have a cervix anymore, we took everything out." That shows you how much we discussed the surgery and alas, how little I knew about my body. I showed her where they resuspend things and asked why they didn't just resuspend the uterus instead of taking it out. She just told me that they didn't do that. She got a little nervous and reminded me that I consented to the surgery.

She then went on vacation, leaving me very worried and upset.

After surgery my bladder wouldn't work, so the nurses would put a catheter in, and when they would take it out, I would bloat up like a whale. So back in it would go. Just before I was to leave the hospital, the doctor who was releasing me informed me that either I would be going home with a Foley catheter, which would be left in all the time, or I could learn to straight catheterize myself on an as needed basis, since my bladder still wasn't working. A nurse came in and took me into the bathroom with a mirror and tried to show me how to straight cath myself, but I was bleeding so badly, I couldn't see to do it. I was also very sore from them putting it in and taking it out over five days. It was very traumatic—here I was, very weak from surgery, standing over the toilet with a straight cath and blood running down my legs and on the floor. I went home with the Foley catheter in.

I never slept well in the hospital, in fact, I barely slept at all. When I got home, it got worse. I could only sleep for 15 to 30 minutes at a time. I started having hot flashes that were so incredible that one-time I even thought I was having a stroke. I remember trying to get upstairs to my sleeping husband, and I had to crawl up the stairs. He got me on the bed and I thought I was going to explode from the heat in me.

When I went back to the doctor the first time, I told her I couldn't sleep,[8] was very sad, and how bad the hot flashes were. She assured me that it was just a matter of adjusting my hormones and doubled my Premarin. I cried a bit and she laughed and said, "Well, I guess we were wrong! Menopause hit you like a Mack truck! Your ovaries must have been working for you to be reacting like this!" Years later, when I got a copy of my records, she indicated I was upset and she "gave me general support."

I was scheduled to come back two weeks after that, but after one week, I didn't feel I was getting better. This was two weeks after surgery, and I was still having bladder trouble. I couldn't pee and had to straight cath myself when my belly would bloat up (actually, my husband helped me with this). I was so constipated if I went once a week (with the help of laxatives) I was pleased. I'd get to the point where I could not eat any more until I had a bowel movement. Then it was so painful, I thought I'd rip everything apart.

My sleeplessness, anxiety, and fatigue had me worried, so I asked my husband to take me to the library. It was the first time I had gotten dressed, other than the doctor visit, and gone out. I took out every book my library had on hysterectomy and menopause. I went home and started reading. I stayed up all night feeling more and more horrified. By the time my husband got up in the morning, I remember screaming at him, "They castrated me!" I was absolutely hysterical and had marked all these pages in the books. They described all the terrible side effects that could occur and the horrible things that could happen. The one thing I remember the most was reading about how they resuspend the vagina where it said—the vagina can fall out, like the finger of a glove. That picture is still with me today and gave me nightmares. I spent another day going over and over the books. I also planned my suicide (pills). However, I knew that I had to confront my doctor first. If I didn't, she'd just keep doing it. My husband called the clinic—he knew something was terribly wrong and took me in. I went in with stacks of books, all marked up with little pieces of paper. I cried and cried and screamed at her. She tried to defend herself at first, then got up and said she was going to "get me help" and that I was not having a "normal reaction" to the surgery.

She called another hospital with a mental health ward, which my husband took me to right away. They took everything away from me, even my shoelaces! The ward was locked and all I did was lay on my bed and cry. I couldn't read, watch TV, or talk. I was only allowed two visitors—my sister and my husband—no phone calls. Every morning at about 6 AM, the psychiatrist would come and we would go in to see him, one by one. He told me I was suffering from hormonal imbalance and sleep deprivation. They started me on drugs to make me sleep right away. I was told I was uncooperative, because in group therapy I wouldn't tell people what was wrong with me. I wanted to scream that I was castrated, but I couldn't say the words. The nurses were told to check on me every 15 to 30 minutes all night long because none of the doctors believed that I didn't sleep at all. They discovered it was true. I didn't sleep at home either, but ever try to sleep in a locked mental ward? There's a lot going on. I finally met with a nurse who got me to talk and said they were going to develop a plan to help me deal with it. My medications were increased daily until the fifth day when I finally slept for two and a half hours. That's how they dealt with it.

Luckily for me on the fifth day, I got a roommate who was crazier than I was. They had tried to keep me in a private room, but the place got too full. When I finally got to sleep for the first time, she kept turning the lights on and making a lot of noise. The next day the psychiatrist said that if I was going to get any sleep, I would have to go home because of her.

I then saw a psychiatrist at first every week, then every two weeks, then once a month. I still cried every time he tried to talk to me. My way of dealing with it was to bury it. His way of dealing with me was to medicate me—with more and more drugs. My whole first year was spent putting one foot in front of the other—just trying to get through my days. After more than a year, he told me he wanted me to see a woman therapist. He felt if I could talk to a woman, it might help me. Once she got me to talk, all I did was cry. Trying to tell my story and how I felt so betrayed by someone I trusted, was so incredibly painful, I could hardly bear it.

I fantasized for months (maybe even years) that my gynecologist got ovarian cancer. It really comforted me. I thought it would be righteous. I went from gynecologist to gynecologist.

My arthritis was horrible. I had dental problems, bladder problems,[3] constipation,[1] hair on my face, but lost it on my head, depression,[9] and brain fog. Some tried to help, but some were just nasty, telling me that none of my problems could be the result of my surgery. I became a great actress, going through all the motions of living. I had two children who needed me. But nothing meant anything to me anymore—not my husband, family or work. I felt lost. I'd find myself approaching a situation and saying to myself, "How would Mary act?" The most frightening times were when I didn't know.

After three years, my insurance changed and I found a new therapist. She was exactly what I needed. She wasn't horrified when she heard how angry I was—she validated my feelings. She taught me to pretend less and to try to live more. I was so lucky to have found her. She had been contemplating a hysterectomy before meeting me, and she said after treating me, she would never consent to it.

I had a weight gain of about 30 pounds,[13] over $3000 worth of dental work in one year, and two cystoscopies because my bladder continued to give me problems. I felt like I was just falling apart. I'd stand in front of the mirror every day, getting ready for work and say, "you fat, ugly, disgusting pig!" (I still do it sometimes). I learned more about my hysterectomy from the urologist who treated me than I did from the doctor who performed it. After only a year and a half, my bladder was already prolapsed a bit. He explained to me that during a vaginal hysterectomy, when the uterus is pulled out, the bladder comes with it. I told him I didn't think mine did, because nobody ever told me that. He said it always happens, because the bladder and uterus are so close together, it isn't possible to get one without the other. He also told me that bladder resuspensions rarely last more than five years. My hysterectomy was in February of 1997. By March 2002, I had to see a doctor because I suspected a prolapsed bladder. She examined me and said I made the right diagnosis, and I needed surgery again to resuspend the bladder. The thought of further surgery made me feel crazy.

My arthritis got so bad after the surgery that I still believe to this day that my ovaries gave me some protection from this disease. I started seeing a rheumatologist who told me I was on his entire arsenal of drugs. I have deformities of my hands and feet. At one point, I was on so many drugs for depression and arthritis, that I'd get up in the morning and just stand in front of all the bottles of pills, feeling very confused. I couldn't remember what to take when. My sister finally made up a chart for me with every day of the week, so all I had to do was look at the day and time. It was a lifesaver.

My marriage suffered terribly and has not recovered. I just lost my feelings for my husband, which was not helped by the fact that sex is not even remotely pleasant for me.[2] I have lumps in my vagina and absolutely no feelings with penetration, except pain occasionally. I was a woman who always had orgasms, from the very first time we had sex. I had three distinct types of orgasms—the best was the "G spot" one. It seems I no longer have a G spot. We went to sex therapy. The therapist told me it was a good thing that sex was 90% in your head. I set her straight on that one. She recommended a vibrator, which I tried. At best, I get a little buzz from it, but it's not like an orgasm, which she assures me it is. Once in a while when it happens, my stomach contracts, which feels very weird and not particularly good. It certainly isn't worth the effort—clipping my toenails or making my grocery list is far more entertaining. I feel like my husband doesn't even try anymore and I am nothing more than an object to be used.

I had a right to know I had other options. I've read some doctors actually do resuspend the uterus. I had a right to know that removing my ovaries was castration and that I could lose my sexuality. I had a right to know there were variations of the surgery. My sex therapist told me that she had just recently had a hysterectomy, but that she "knew enough to keep her cervix and ovaries." Even then, she admitted that sex was not like it used to be. I had a right to know about HRT and the risks associated with it. I had a right to have the opportunity to make an INFORMED CONSENT.

Having said that, I don't know if I will ever forgive myself for not thoroughly investigating it before I had it done. Many of my "happy hysterectomy" friends now admit to many of the same problems I have. Some still deny it. My favorite is the friend who had a hysterectomy in her 30s and has said she doesn't care if she ever has sex again—but it's NOT because of her surgery— her doctor assured her of that. Too many women parrot what their doctors tell them—and it's almost always "that has nothing to do with the surgery," or they imply it's all in your head.

I'm no longer on anti-depressants now. I finally just took myself off them. I figured this is my life now and I'd better learn to deal with it. It is pathetic how our society positively reveres a man's sexuality and will do anything to preserve it—Viagra, penile implants, nerve grafts, etc. Yet, this same medical profession sees no problem with the wholesale castration of women. What doctor would dare castrate a man? Women are told directly and indirectly that our sexuality is not important. As long as the vagina is still there, for the man's use, you are considered "fine." If you complain, they tell you that just being close is more important. Tell that to a man! This unconscionable treatment of women by the medical profession must be stopped. Isn't there a societal impact on extending and preserving our husband's sex lives, while doctors are castrating their wives?

I investigated suing the doctor who performed my surgery, but by the time I was out of my drug-induced stupor enough to consider it, the statute of limitations had nearly run out, and it just wasn't possible to get a case together. I've written to many magazines, TV talk shows, and lots of Internet sites—screaming to be heard. Maybe some women do feel better after, but for me it's a nightmare that will never end. I even wrote my doctor, 2 1/2 years after the surgery. It was a scathing letter detailing my suffering and her ineptitude. I told her she was a poor excuse for a doctor. The head of the clinic wrote me back a very condescending letter saying they were sorry I was feeling poorly, and if I would come back to the clinic they would see how they could help me. Yeah, right—what body parts do they want now? Since they can't give me my life (or my uterus) back, I never bothered.

I have always felt that part of the reason for my prolapsed uterus was that when I had my first child I was in labor for 26 hours. My own doctor had to leave hours into my labor because he had a vacation trip planned. I was left in the care of the on-call doctor that night. We live in a small town outside of a major metro area. As it happened, during the time I was in labor, ten women delivered—a daunting task for one doctor, I'm sure. However, when I was wheeled into delivery, the doctor immediately told me he was going to use forceps because I was too worn out to help with the pushing. I begged my husband to talk him out of it, but he did it anyway. Immediately after the birth of my child, the doctor wrapped the cord around the forceps and yanked the afterbirth out of me. I started bleeding so bad, my husband nearly fainted. He saw it and told me what the doctor did. We had gone to childbirth classes and knew that was not supposed to happen. I figure this doctor was so exhausted that he just didn't care (I was the last one of the ten women to deliver). I was not allowed to hold my child, I vaguely remember everybody around me and I kept asking for my baby. Later, they brought my son to me in my room, I had lost so much valuable bonding time with him, and I was very distressed about it. I asked the nurse why I couldn't have had him right away and why nobody would answer my questions about his well-being. She said, "We were far more worried about the mother, than the baby." Apparently, the doctor's actions caused so much bleeding that they were trying to decide whether or not I needed a transfusion. It was well into the next day, before they decided that they would hold off (I never did get one). For a couple of weeks after delivery, large chunks of bloody mass would come out when I went to the bathroom—I'm talking the size of a large orange or small grapefruit. I never had any such problem after the birth of my second child.

I also want to pass this along, if men had babies, this sort of thing would never happen. What made me think of it again, is that I went to the urology surgeon this week and her first question was, "Did I ever have a forceps delivery?" She also told me the surgery I need is vaginal and I freaked. I told her I wanted no more vaginal surgery because the hysterectomy destroyed my nerves. She replied that nerve damage in vaginal hysterectomy is well-documented, but that the type of surgery she was recommending affects an area which is known to have fewer nerves and that most women do not have problems with it.

—Mary - St. Paul, Minnesota USA

Writer's Profile

ಚಿಚಿಚಿಚಿಚಿಚಿಚಿಚಿಚಿಚಿ   ಜುಜುಜುಜುಜುಜುಜುಜುಜುಜು

Authored by:	Debbie
Age:	44
From:	Oakdale, Minnesota USA
Hysterectomy:	1998
Age at surgery	39
2 Ovaries removed	1998
Age at surgery	39
Reason for surgery/surgeries:	Erroneously performed due to malfunctioning gallbladder
Hormone replacement history:	1998 to present Bi-est sublingual
Other medications:	Zoloft® (anti-depressant)

In 1998 I was castrated, because of a bad gallbladder . . . and a bad doctor . . . and very bad timing. I was 39 years old, married, and the mother of two. I had just begun a career in real estate, realizing a ten-year dream of mine. It was exciting, I was good at it, and my earning potential was limitless. I was living the American dream.

In March, I entered a hospital for abdominal pain, which I'd been having for a week or so with increasing pain and frequency. While I'd had no history of any gynecological problems, I did have one laparoscopy to remove adhesions which had grown after my two cesareans. Not a gynecological disorder, mind you, simply a post-surgical malady that occurs frequently in both men and women. Because that was the only health issue I'd ever encountered, it was suspected that perhaps those adhesions had returned. I spent the night in the hospital and the next day I met the ob-gyn who was on the surgery schedule for that day. Having never before met this doctor, I knew nothing about him and he knew nothing about me. He had an opening available and had scheduled me for a laparoscopy. However, when I indicated to him that the location of my pain was high up in the abdomen, around the sternum area, we thought that perhaps something else was to blame here. He called in an internal medicine doctor, who performed upper abdominal ultrasounds to check for gallstones. Although no gallstones were evident, I later learned that typically one out of five gallbladder patients have no gallstones whatsoever.

The laparoscopy remained scheduled for that afternoon. I was brought down to the "holding area" outside the operating room. I was given something to relax me from the anesthesiologist. A nurse brought in a consent form for me to sign. It contained the words "laparoscopy, laparotomy, and hysterectomy, if necessary." I asked that nurse why hysterectomy was on there. The doctor certainly had never mentioned this to me. We were just doing a laparoscopy. She replied, "Oh well, we always put that in there as a matter of procedure . . . you know . . . in case they should get in there and find something." Not sure what that "something" was, but thinking of malignancy, I signed. Later, another nurse returned with two additions to the consent form. They were "appendectomy and BSO" (bilateral salpingo-oophorectomy: removal of both fallopian tubes and ovaries). I did not know what BSO meant, but assumed it had something to do with appendectomy. I wondered if I was supposed to sign the form or initial it. She told me to initial it.

When I awoke in the recovery room, I heard the surgeon's assistant tell me, "Deborah, we took out your uterus and both your ovaries. Now you'll never have to worry about uterine cancer or ovarian cancer." I couldn't open my eyes or speak, but I felt a single tear running down my cheek. It was the first of many.

The following day, my surgeon came in to tell me that he thought he had found some very minor, fresh endometriosis. He matter-of-factly mentioned that he wasn't positive this was the right surgery, but felt it probably was. In any event, he would put an estrogen patch on me and I'd feel just the same as I did before the surgery.

I was filled with many questions. How was this surgery performed? How were my ovaries taken out? Did I still have a cervix? What about this patch? Where do I put it? He hurriedly answered these questions and told me I should return to work in two weeks because the quicker I went back to work, the quicker I could forget about this whole thing.

I wondered how I could forget that I no longer had my reproductive organs? Hysterectomy is derived from the word hysteria. I now know why.

Within weeks, I discovered I was unable to tolerate the estrogen patch due to severe calf pain reminiscent of the phlebitis I experienced while on birth control pills years before. Also, my abdominal pain was returning . . . big time. A nuclear scan showed that my gallbladder was not properly functioning and that it, too, needed to be removed. This was just weeks after my hysterectomy. Because I'd had to remove my estrogen patch, I was now in full-blown surgical menopause. My hair was falling out and turning gray (in all areas), my scalp bled from the sudden loss of hormones, my pelvic area was so inflamed, I was tested for a bladder infection (negative), and my heart palpitations were coming on so heavy and strong I remember checking my chest to see if it was bruised. I couldn't sit up for more than a few minutes due to crushing fatigue and weakness. I couldn't think straight or track information. I was so dizzy, even pouring a glass of milk without spilling was nearly impossible. What was happening to me?

My life had gone suddenly insane as the trauma of my situation set in. How could this have happened? How could this have happened TO ME?

I was determined to keep my six-week post-op checkup with the surgeon who'd done this to me. I found out my pathology report was perfectly clear. My intent was to tell this crazy butcher he'd done the wrong operation! My hope, however, was that he'd tell me this hysterectomy was warranted, and that I most certainly had needed it—anything to make me feel there was a reason for this hell I was living in. Instead, the exact opposite happened. He lied and said another doctor had phoned him at home and told him there was a hysterectomy patient waiting for him. When I told him that just couldn't be true, he spun his story around again. I suddenly saw this man for what he was . . . a liar.

I went home and went to bed—for the next 14 months. During that time, I tried every synthetic estrogen known . . . all with debilitating side effects. My limbs always had veinous inflammatory responses . . . calves and feet, forearms and hands. I felt as though I had electrical voltages shooting throughout my extremities! It was a shooting, searing, burning pain. I couldn't sit or stand still. The pain was torturous . . . and nobody could help me. I went from doctor to doctor searching for help—but there was none. I learned about compounded estrogens and compounding pharmacies from a local TV newscast. Alarmed, I phoned my latest ob-gyn to request a prescription. She supposedly knew so much about HRT, yet she'd told me all estrogens were basically the same. I realize now what a ridiculous statement that was. It's like saying all humans are basically the same! Why then would some people be allergic to penicillin and others not? My reactions to all synthetic estrogens were "toxic." When I began taking compounded estrogens, the burning was alleviated, but my many other symptoms were not.

Four years have passed since my hysterectomy and oophorectomy. I have lost my business that I once loved and worked so hard at. I am, as one doctor referred to me, "a hysterectomy cripple." I have constant tingling, numbness and parasthesias in my hands, forearms, calves, and feet, which makes it difficult to sit with both feet on the floor—I must keep them elevated. I've been diagnosed with peripheral neuropathy (nerve damage), possible reflex sympathetic dystrophy (RSD), fibromyalgia (a very common side effect to this surgery), and a malaligned pelvis. I have much trunk pain, hip pain, and lower back pain. I have short-term memory lapses,[6] and still experience much fatigue.

When I dream at night, I become the healthy, vibrant woman I used to be. There is no pain in my dreams. But then of course, I must wake up . . . to the chronic pain, which serves as a reminder to me of all that has happened . . . and all that could have been . . . if only . . .

—Debbie - Oakdale, Minnesota USA

Writer's Profile

ՃՑՃՑՃՑՃՑՃՑՃՑՃՑՃՑՃՑ   ՑՄՑՄՑՄՑՄՑՄՑՄՑՄՑՄՑՄՑՄ

Authored by: Olivia Dresher
Age: 56
From: Seattle, Washington USA

Hysterectomy: 1994
Age at surgery   49

2 Ovaries removed   1994
Age at surgery   49

Reason for
    surgery/surgeries: Fibroids (extreme bleeding)

Hormone replacement
    history: 1995 to 2000
                          Creams, pills, and patches

Other medications: Not reported

I had my surgery over seven years ago, when I was 49 years old. My uterus, ovaries, and cervix were removed by abdominal incision. I had small fibroids, but they caused near-constant bleeding and intermittent hemorrhaging. I actively tried to avoid major surgery for almost a year, using both conventional and alternative medicine. The hysterectomy was a last resort. I had lost a lot of weight from the worry and stress of unpredictable hemorrhaging. However, the surgery created many new problems that have never been resolved, no matter how many doctors I've consulted.

My notebooks are filled with many thoughts and feelings about the aftermath of this surgery. The first two years post hysterectomy I felt I had lost my essence, and through my writing I expressed and tried to understand the strange new country I lived in. Today, I don't feel that I've *lost* my essence, but that I'm missing some *color* of my essence.

What follows are journal fragments that date back to 1995-1996 (one to two years after my surgery). They capture the tone of my outer struggle, as it mingled with my inner struggle. When I re-read these fragments now, I see how deeply I still feel this way. However, I don't fall into the post-surgery despair as much as I used to. My symptoms, now, have been more integrated into my life, even though they have never gone away, and new ones still appear. The following are excerpts from my journal entries.

August 14, 1995

What's horrifying is to watch the transformation that's going on, for every day I get further and further away from the person I was. I can't dance with my life anymore; now my life is a detour filled with obstacles, and I react extremely, because I can't handle anything. I yell, I wince, I pace, I sigh.

As I was walking home alone last night in the dark, the street lights went out as I passed under them. It became so dark I could hardly see, but I kept walking. I was getting close to home, when suddenly I thought we were having a huge earthquake.

My whole body felt pushed back and forth, and I felt the sidewalk underneath me fall like an elevator going down. Suddenly it was as if I was under water, too, because I couldn't hear. To keep myself from falling, I held on to the nearest tree. I looked up at what I *could* see (telephone wires, tree branches), wondering if anything else was shaking. But no, it wasn't an earthquake, it was just me, a self-quake. After several minutes, I was able to walk again, but whatever I had just experienced disturbed me because it made me realize how *total* an internal reality can be, how it can radically change the way I experience *external* reality.

<u>August 16, 1995</u>

Every day there are new symptoms, or variations on the already many current symptoms. V's way of responding to this is to ask me, "What's the symptom-of-the-day, what's the pain-of-the-week?" I laugh, wishing laughter truly could heal, wishing I could make myself laugh when I'm alone.

I'm edging towards the conclusion (and edging toward accepting the conclusion) that I might never be well again, that this might be a steady decline. Is there no hope, is that what I need to face? Now that I no longer dance with my life, do I need to learn how to dance with death? First the bleeding wouldn't go away, and now the pains and symptoms post-bleeding won't go away. Nothing goes away anymore.

<u>August 20, 1995</u>

Who is this person I've become? Even her habits aren't mine. I'm trying to live with her. I'm trying to let her fill the space that has been empty ever since the old self was forced out.

<u>August 28, 1995</u>

I'm beginning to feel that I dreamed up who I used to be. Sexuality, especially, feels like a dream.[2] The whole landscape of self has changed, and my old self is extinct. I feel that my "new" self is just a small and hintful version of what I once was—like comparing a lizard to a brontosaurus. My old self came from another time and place; my new self breathes in dusty memories of my old self, and coughs. The new and the old don't get along. I keep trying to build a bridge between the two, but the ever present storms keep washing the bridge away. I spend so much energy building bridges that never last. To give up, though, would be to throw myself into a tidal wave.

August 29, 1995

The anniversary of my surgery—and I have a doctor's appointment today, but these appointments are beginning to feel futile. Doctors stare at me as if I'm making up or exaggerating my symptoms, as if my problems are *psychological* because the suggestions and treatments I keep trying do not help me.

September 2, 1995

My body is a mountain that I'm climbing. I'm weary from the aches of the climb. My body has become mystical to me—a terrible mystery. My body is also a tent, pseudo shelter, offering no real protection from the extreme temperatures outside. The soul longs to soar; but my body traps my soul, stuffs it inside, keeps it in chains. My soul is drowning in my body. My life, under the surface, is a life lived while drowning. I snap and have no patience with the mundane details, because air is too precious to waste. I am both the mountain *and* the body that's climbing the mountain.

But my body is not a "body." My body is this "I," this "me"— longing for release.

September 3, 1995

As I write this, I don't trust my body. I don't trust my heart racing and skipping beats. I don't trust the pains in my legs (so intense I can't even bend down). I don't trust the feeling that I can't breathe fully. I don't trust the painful spasms in my bladder, or the ringing in my ears. I don't trust the surgery incision that still swells up, red, and sore.

I remember the 10 year old Olivia, and feel a horror having to tell her that this is what her life has turned out to be. I have to break the news to her that nothing ever worked out, her dreams remained miracles that never happened, and her life ended up this way. I take her in my arms and tell her this, and we cry together, rock together, sway and say no words at all after I tell her.

September 4, 1995

So I'll never be the same again. So I might have to live with symptoms always—they might never go away. These thoughts have become the main theme of my life, the melody that keeps replaying and repeating. I'm letting it, because I *am* it. I'm this melody of symptoms. Nobody wants to know this. Nobody sees me for what I've become. I don't lament this—I just notice. The melody, the melody, at least it *is* a melody.

When I see doctors, I get the feeling that I'm not supposed to ask questions—not supposed to have unexplainable symptoms. How odd that I keep going to doctors. I don't even trust western medicine, and yet I'm full of despair from all these tests. My blood, my saliva, my stools—everything—has been tested and retested.

September 7, 1995

To live in health would be ecstasy. To not have weird symptoms, to not have pain, to not have to have countless tests and doctor appointments, and empty speculations about what's wrong (and why) would be ecstasy. To not have to *pretend* to be well would be ecstasy. To not have to *worry* about the body would be ecstasy. But the days of health are probably over for me. I'm simply grateful that things aren't worse. I'm grateful as long as I can still walk and see and hear and do what means most to me. I'm grateful as long as literature, and music, and nature can be my life. I'm grateful for this very moment that I'm writing in this journal. I'm grateful to be able to hear and love the music on the radio. I'm grateful to be in this house, smelling the air outside through the open window, and watching the sun peeking through the clouds. I'm grateful for the wildlife that visits my backyard. I'm grateful for being able to walk outside in the morning, and

finding breakfast on the fruit trees. I'm grateful that I can still
be grateful, in spite of everything.

September 9, 1995

In my body I live in another time and place. I no longer
live in the 20th century. The intense aches in my legs and hands
feel mysterious; there is no name for what's happening to me. I
am declining, it seems, from deep inside, as if it's 1800 (when
people declined in pain and mystery). The woman next door
asks me how I am, saying I look fine. "Fine," I agree (tired of
revealing that I am *not* fine). "Fine," I say again in return, as if
I'm just saying "hi," and then I walk away with intense pain in
every leg muscle, hating the truths that can't be told, expressed,
or embraced.

October 12, 1995

What is wrong with my body? Is it true that surgery
permanently altered it, and nothing can be done now? Am I
having problems because nerves were severed, scar tissue is taking
over, and the colon/bladder area has been so rearranged that
nothing works smoothly anymore? Am I having problems
because what they removed from me was the very link to my
well-being?

This body is not fully mine anymore. It has become a tumor
growing out of my spirit. It's an alien from another planet that
the doctors have no idea what to do with.

I try to live—and most everyone thinks I'm okay—but I'm
in a web, an insect caught in the spider's trap. My spirit is that
insect, and my body is the spider that devours it.

October 25, 1995

Half the day is spent dealing with the weirdnesses of my
body. It takes me hours to prepare to even go outside. I never
know how bad it's going to get. The pain. I have no control over
my body. There is always the fear of another emergency, and
that I will end up in the hospital again. That's my *worst* fear.

October 26, 1995

Now I imagine health to be the greatest luxury, yet I really can't even *imagine* health anymore. I keep going from doctor to doctor, but my symptoms remain out there somewhere, unfathomable.

And so, yes, I imagine—if I *could* imagine it—that health is the greatest luxury. To not have to *worry* about the body would be the greatest luxury. To have the simple solutions *work* would be the luxury.

Taking a bath this afternoon, after talking with one of my doctors on the phone for 20 minutes, I cried and cried for the first time in months. Wails without tears as I took a bath. How strange that there were no tears (lack of tears: another post-surgery symptom for me). I cried into the hopelessness of my body, the hopelessness of all my trying. Crying tear less tears in a clawfoot tub.

November 1, 1995

A few months after the surgery, a small shadow of my sexuality was left, a faint glow. But now not even *that* remains, and the shadow has left only a brief outline of what was, and even *that* seems to be disappearing. More and more there's just physical pain and emptiness where once there was ecstasy and worlds within worlds. As if the death of sexuality says: *you better start facing the bigger death yet to come! Let this first death teach you well and guide you.* But teach me *what*—to find a part of whatever I am that has nothing to do with the physical body? I still love intensely, and the same longing for intimacy exists, but sexuality as I knew it has vanished. I'm like a blind person trying to see colors, or a deaf person trying to hear music. Secretly I imagine inventing new ways to be sexual, but who will join me there? There's a sad desolate peace in this loss.

December 18, 1995

I can't even remember what my intense sexuality was like. I find that very strange—that I can't close my eyes and at least *remember* the way I used to feel. I try, but I only feel my present state—these wounds, scars, and the emptiness. But tonight on the radio a slow guitar song was playing, and suddenly I felt a stab of feeling like the old sensations, sweet and sharp, and memories of my first year in Seattle were brought back instantly. Not sexual memories/feelings, specifically, but memories of the wide, rich quality of feeling that I used to carry around with me when I *was* sexual. But within a minute the feeling was gone, like a mirage.

January 5, 1996

In trying to get better, it's almost the feeling of trying to grow back an arm or a leg. It's so obvious to me that the surgery has caused severe structural alterations deep inside, no matter *what* doctors say or don't say. So the question is now: "*How* do I learn to live without an arm or a leg?"

Where's the person/doctor who can help me? Does such a person/doctor even exist? Looking for a doctor is as futile as looking for love. I need a doctor who has no preconceived notions about what a woman might be experiencing. Someone who will really explore my various symptoms. Someone who views the body as sacred. Someone who isn't in it for the money. Someone who loves. Someone who isn't dogmatic. Someone who knows that hysterectomy can cause many problems. Someone who is determined to find an explanation that's *true*. (*I* should be that doctor; if only I *could* be—for myself first, and then for others.)

January 23, 1996

To have so many symptoms and to not know what's wrong, or why the symptoms persist in spite of treatment, is crazy-making. It's like being in a foreign country where no one speaks your language and you have no map, no place to stay, and so you just wonder and wander. It's like living in one of Kafka's nightmares.

It's not that I try to distract myself from my physical symptoms in order to live my life, but that the symptoms keep trying to distract *me* from all I long to do. But, I never give in to not being well; I always resist, but hence, I'm never whole—to resist is to be fragmented.

July 27, 1996

It has been almost two years since the surgery. I keep hoping my body will bounce back, but it just *doesn't* bounce back. I simply have a different body now, a flawed and weakened body with eccentric symptoms, and that's the way it is. I need to embrace this, and travel on with this new reality, not always try to travel back to the old reality. I need to embrace the many symptoms, including the unpredictable moments of intense pain when I come close to fainting. I need to embrace the symptoms as a whole, as a chorus singing to me that I will listen to, no longer obsessed with the separate voices. I need to embrace this chorus of symptoms.

—Olivia Dresher - Seattle, Washington USA

Writer's Profile

ଓଓଓଓଓଓଓଓଓଓଓଓ ଯଯଯଯଯଯଯଯଯଯଯ

Authored by:	Lorrie W.
Age:	46
From:	Orange County, California USA
Hysterectomy:	1999
Age at surgery	42
2 Ovaries removed	1999
Age at surgery	42
Reason for surgery/surgeries:	Multiple symptoms, excessive bleeding, cysts, and pain
Hormone replacement history:	1999 to present Estrace® (oral estradiol)
Other medications:	None

I am now 46 years old, Caucasian, born and raised in Southern California where I have lived my entire life, except for a five year period when I lived in California's Central Valley.

I have had "female problems" since I began menstruating at the age of 11. From the very beginning, my very erratic periods were a nightmare—heavy bleeding, clotting, horrid cramps, nausea, painful breasts, etc. I often had to stay in bed the first day or two of each period. Throughout each cycle I went through a roller coaster of extreme emotional states, much to the dismay of those around me.

This continued until I was 18, and I was put on birth control pills. Finally, some relief! It brought most of my symptoms under some control. When I was 22, I went off the pill and had my daughter on my 23rd birthday. My pregnancy was dreadful. I was sick as a dog all day, every day, from when I got pregnant until daughter's birth.

I tried to stay off birth control pills for a couple more years, but due to the increasing severity of symptoms, went back on them and continued to take them until the age of 42 (when I had my hysterectomy).

Over the years my symptoms increased and worsened in severity. I began suffering from internal benign cysts—on my ovaries, fallopian tubes, bladder, uterus, etc. They were very painful. Some of the cysts dissipated or burst on their own (hellish moments) and some had to be surgically removed through laparoscopy. I also experienced a terribly painful condition called mittelschmerz syndrome (ovulation pain), with the frequency of occurrences increasing over the years.

As I approached the age of 40, the problems continued to worsen, including weight gain. Finally, in March of 1999, at the ripe old age of 42, I had a total hysterectomy—uterus, tubes and ovaries. The doctor discussed all aspects with me very thoroughly and gently. He was very compassionate, knowledgeable and professional. The day of the surgery I was put on 1 mg of estrogen daily.

It has now been about four years since the most heavenly day of my life. My postoperative recovery was far less miserable than my menstrual cycles had been! My physical symptoms have disappeared, sex is no longer painful,[2] and my emotional state is steady and pleasant. I still smile smugly every time I pass the feminine hygiene section at the store, and think how terrific it is that I no longer have to deal with those problems.

The only negative has been a lot of weight gain since the surgery, despite improved nutrition and exercise routines. While I have struggled hard to lose the weight, it is still a small price to pay for the glorious benefits I continue to enjoy after my surgery. I consider the day of my hysterectomy to be the day that, after 31 years, I was finally liberated from the hell of being female.

—Lorrie W. - Orange Country, California USA

Writer's Profile

ෞෞෞෞෞෞෞෞෞෞෞ   ෨ෞ෨ෞ෨ෞ෨ෞ෨ෞ෨ෞ

Authored by:	Grace
Age:	45
From:	Maine USA
Hysterectomy:	2001
Age at surgery	43
2 Ovaries removed	2001
Age at surgery	43
Reason for surgery/surgeries:	Conization complications, after CIN II Pap smear, resulting in uterine blockage leading to pelvic inflammatory disease, and potential uterine rupture
Hormone replacement history:	2001 to present Vivelle® patch, testosterone and progesterone cream
Other medication:	Bupropion (anti-depressant)

In January 2001, I found myself in what appeared to be a life-or-death situation, with the only remedy being a hysterectomy. In the months that followed, I felt as though I indeed had died, and still continue to have haunting concerns about my health, and life in general.

I have spent much time going over all prior medical interventions, and influences. I have looked for anything that I could have changed that led to me being in the position where I had to allow a surgeon to remove beloved organs, which I had battled for years to sustain and keep.

In 1987, at age 29, after having my regular gynecologic exam, I received a letter telling me that I had a positive Pap smear, and that I was being referred to a surgical associate. I called the practice for information, and to ask why something as alarming as a positive Pap smear was communicated to me in a letter. I was told they were "unable to reach me by phone," although I had a functional answering machine.

When I went to the doctor, the nurse showed me pictures of cone biopsies. The doctor's manner was brusque and sharp, quite the opposite of my compassionate gynecologist. She performed a preliminary punch biopsy, and as tears ran down my face, her nurse, who did not stop chattering through my procedure, joked that "you must be premenstrual!" (because I expressed a normal emotion at the time). I trusted the women's health care facility I chose, and I did not expect to have to guard myself for insensitivity, miscommunications, and other negligences. I received a call telling me that I had CIN II, and that I would need a cone biopsy.

I called my gynecologist to ask her for any alternatives? She looked up my smear, and told me that it was normal, and any irregularities " must be a sign of the harmonic convergence." (I was aware of the harmonic convergence occurring at this time in August 1987, but didn't get her point. However, based on this response I didn't pursue continued medical care with her.)

I ended up going to a gynecologist that a friend of the family worked for. I had never had serious gynecologic problems prior to this positive Pap smear, and lacked the experience and relentless searching capacity that I now possess for locating competent health practitioners.

This older male gynecologist, who claimed I had cervical intraepithelial neoplasia II (CIN II) from the human papilloma virus, which came from "playing house" (!), gave me, what I learned later was a radical conization. He also made toxic and judgmental comments and inferences about my sexuality. At the time, I happened to be divorcing and emerging from an unhealthy marriage (for all I know, the positive Pap smear results could have been a manifestation of the violation I experienced during this married period).

After my conization, my biopsy results revealed that my tissues evidenced no CIN III, just some CIN I, and cellular irregularities.

Later physicians remarked that my cervical area looked "maimed," "mauled," or actually said, "where your cervix USED to be," leading me to question the necessity of such an aggressive cone. I was told by some that they rarely saw such a dramatic conization (some would cringe upon first examining me), and Pap smears became very, very difficult to perform, since there was no cervical tissue left to take the smear from.

Three years after my surgery, I experienced severe abdominal pains and fever, and was hospitalized. My current gynecologist had gone out of practice due to health problems, so I met and worked with another gynecologist in his practice. He told me that I had a huge ovarian abscess, and was in the "96% mortality range for women, should the fluid-filled mass burst." I was placed on maximum IV antibiotics for ten days, then released, continuing on oral antibiotics for months. He recommended that I stay on birth control pills, explaining that the cervix is a protective gateway for the reproductive system. It secretes uterine-protecting mucus, etc. He stated that since I had no cervix left, I would always be at risk of developing abscesses, pelvic inflammatory disease (PID), etc., just from the NORMAL BACTERIA THAT EXISTS IN THE VAGINA alone.

I tried being on the pill, and could not bear the side effects and the feelings of strained abnormality (now that I understand natural HRT, I know why). My reality was continually questioned, rather than affirmed, because I could not tolerate the pill, thus, a crucial health care provider was unfortunately distanced.

I had a laparoscopy later that year to check the health of my organs—the doctor removed endometriosis, and repaired one ovary and scarred fallopian tubes. I experienced pain with intercourse in the ovary area continuously after that. Two years later, another laparotomy was performed to allow for more extensive removal of adhesions.

Continual follow-ups and ultrasounds showed that my organs appeared healthy. My periods were always regular and felt very cleansing. I believe in the spiritual qualities of the "blood mysteries" and honored my body's ability to cleanse and renew itself through the menstrual cycles.

By 1997, I started having more pain with intercourse and unusually heavy cramping with the onset of periods, so I visited my doctor. He said that since I wasn't on the pill, I continued to be at risk for intense internal infections, and that progressive hormonal changes would cause intensified menstrual problems. He said that he couldn't keep "patching me up" and that he was recommending a hysterectomy by age 45 (I was 39 at the time).

I spent the following years investing great focus and conscious action in preventing this outcome. I studied Qi Gong with a brilliant Chinese physician, worked with a naturopath to strengthen my immune system and balance my reproductive organs, did a cleanse for years that involved eating only the cleanest natural food (which I have continued), exercised diligently, had a reading with a medical intuitive who told me "even if all my reproductive organs were removed, my pelvis would still resonate with trauma." I worked on the therapeutic level to address trauma, as well as consulted with other gynecologists who were said to have strong reputations.

In 1998, I became very concerned because I became completely disabled with pelvic pain at the onset of every period, as well as at other times during the month. One of the general practitioners who was covering for my general practitioner told me I had irritable bowel syndrome (a dangerous misdiagnosis, I later discovered). I consulted with another doctor who told me it was probably endometriosis, to take Motrin, and live with it. By 2000, I became aware that my intense pain was due to blockage—my uterus was battling to dispel blood, but the opening was essentially blocked where my cervix once was. After days of disabling pain, aspirin, and castor oil packs, my period would finally flood through a uterine opening described as ordinarily having the visible width of a pinhole.

I searched for a physician who would surgically open up the cervical passage. However, my general practitioner's referral thought that if I used Premarin cream internally, it would help to open the base of the uterus, and facilitate menstrual flow. I felt terrible on Premarin, like a frenzied pregnant mare (I was not aware of what Premarin was composed of at the time), and discontinued that. This was the autumn of 2000—I went back to the doctor because the intense pelvic pain was continuous. He told me he would book a laparoscopy for the spring, and attempt to open the cervical uterine area then. He thought my pain was due to endometriosis.

Then two years ago, on December 27, 2000, I began to have intense abdominal pain. I had tried to prepare for this menstrual period by taking aspirin for days before (I had reactions to Motrin). My pain intensified. I called the gynecologist on New Year's Eve and cried in pain and despair. He overlooked prospects of uterine blockage, said that "endometriosis is a debilitating condition," and advised me to continue over the counter pain medications and come to his office during the beginning of the week.

My abdomen swelled, the agonizing pain continued. I could not stand up straight, eat, or function. One of my friends visited me and was shocked because I looked so terrible and deathly. I called another gynecologist's office to consult with and make an appointment with a female doctor about whom I had heard good things. She prescribed a heavy pain medication over the phone, which did not touch the pain.

As soon as her office was open, she accepted me for an appointment. She felt a big mass in the cervical area, and a big ovarian mass. I had an ultrasound, which confirmed both masses, but the technician was puzzled at the odd, large mass near the bottom of the uterus.

The doctor advised a hysterectomy, and removal of my often infected ovary. After being so weakened and sick, I did not see any alternatives. She said she would try to save the other ovary, if possible.

My pain quieted down on January 7 (surgery was scheduled for January 9). I was relaxing with a friend that evening, and suddenly a huge amount of blood was released, a literal bloodbath. The doctor told me that it sounded like a "decompression" and not to worry. I was very weak, but not in pain by the time I went in for surgery.

I awoke to be told that both ovaries had to be taken. The non-infected one had an endometrioma (a non-cancerous mass of endometrial tissue and blood), and I was told its survival would not have been promising. There were many adhesions in my pelvis that required much time and effort to remove. After awakening, I had a massive "burned at the stake" hot flash, for which I received an estradiol patch.

The intern-in-training told me that there had been a rupture from the blood-filled uterus through the vaginal wall, but later denied telling me this. Months later, I discovered a bump in my vagina—when I went in to have that checked, the physician told me that was where the mass of blood in the distorted uterus had ruptured through the vaginal wall in order to discharge—that had been the "cervical mass" seen in the ultrasound. In much simpler terms, my blocked cervical opening prevented me from bleeding normally, and created the conditions for massive internal infection, right ovary mass, distended, inflamed fallopian tubes, severe adhesions, high fever, chills, severe pain . . . all seriously threatening physical conditions. My ovaries had apparently worked valiantly through all the prior infections, as was evidenced by regular and blocked, but otherwise healthy periods.

I intensely regret not asking to view my removed reproductive organs after surgery. Although they may not have looked pretty, if I had had the opportunity to see them looking diseased, I would have felt more acceptance about having them removed. Also, I wish I had viewed them to allow myself to say good-bye to a crucial and inestimateably valuable part of my body, which I literally experienced attunement and rhythm through. At the time, I lacked the energy and consciousness to advocate and assert for what could have been regarded as an odd and troublesome request.

Less than two weeks after surgery, I experienced massive tooth pain, and had to have a root canal. At the same time, my significant other, with whom I had experienced a very sexually passionate relationship, sent me an e-mail telling me that he did not wish to remain involved with me.

In the months following surgery, I went through terrible side effects—intense palpitations, hot flashes, sweats, and much crying. I tried to separate the kinds of grieving I was experiencing from the hormonal side effects, and was challenged with that. I missed three months from work due to the wrenching side effects. Shortly after surgery, I entered weekly therapy, and began acupuncture to help me resume sleeping and balance. The acupuncture was immediately effective at calming my enervated system and allowing me to rest. The acupuncturist had undergone a hysterectomy herself (no oophorectomy), and was compassionate and knowing.

I began using Vivelle 1 mg patch after surgery (January 2001), but still had severe palpitations, sweats, hot flashes, mood swings, etc. I researched compounded creams, met with a compounding pharmacist, and was put on compounded bi-est, progesterone, and testosterone (February 2001). Unfortunately, the bi-est did not stay in my system consistently and I continued to have intense palpitations. So, because it could not provide me with regularity, I had to replace bi-est with the Vivelle patch (April 2001). I continued to have side effects. It was suspected that I had "estrogen dominance," and my estrogen patch was lowered to .075 mg.

I was on Vivelle 0.075 mg until November of 2002. It was then upped to the 1 mg strength, which I am currently on. I was on progesterone 1 mg (100 mg per gram) and testosterone 0.25 mg (1 mg per gram) until August 2002. My hot flashes and palpitations diminished for a while, but by the summer of 2002, I still had constant intense fatigue and inertia, and was losing massive amounts of hair.

After testing, my progesterone levels were found to be very, very high, contributing to an androgen build-up, and I was advised to discontinue both progesterone and testosterone. I had begun to see a menopause expert, and a key advisor regarding hormone replacement—she helped to guide me in dosage decisions for hormone replacement.

I continued to experience exhaustion, depression, and flatness, and finally decided to request antidepressants in November.[9] I am trying Bupropion, which has been somewhat of a stimulant, but I know that the lack of testosterone and progesterone (which I am beginning to resume), as well as the lack of all the real things that my body so beautifully produced, has been leaving my life deficient—and feeling very desolate.

I had one brief relationship last year, which was a godsend in the respect that I learned I can still experience some pleasure with intimacy and intercourse. I have not had an orgasm with a partner, however, since surgery. I greatly lack drive for exercise, sexual connection,[2] and often just play and fun, in general. The words "fixed" and "neutered" come to mind as I try to express how I feel now.

I lost the back grinding tooth that I had to have the root canal on two weeks after surgery, and am now looking at the prospects of losing the opposite grinding tooth, even after very expensive crown and root canal work.

I just had a polysomnogram (assessment of possible biological causes of sleep disorders) to rule out sleep disorder as relating to my fatigue.[8] I will be going on my follow-up visit shortly.

I was told I need surgery for the distorting bunions on both feet (my feet muscles have contracted since surgery). I am allaying that for the time being with orthopedic inserts.

I have had to have my contact lenses changed four times in less than two years due to the rapid eye changes I am experiencing. My breast mass is diminished (I had a slender, athletic build, but still "used" to have breasts, and a proportionate figure).

On a bright note, I was happy to learn that my bone density test last summer showed me to have "the bones of a young woman" (two family members have early osteoporosis). Now, however, I wonder about the long term forecast.

I have tried to live with my decision for the complete hysterectomy, believing that I did not have many options at the time. I experience this surgery as a daily loss, right down to the feelings of cold scar tissue and physical emptiness in my pelvis, and the feeling that my vagina drops lower if I move or try to dance. I feel I am experiencing an acceleration in aging, thinning hair going white, and physical pain, which I now recognize as fibromyalgia.

I am trying not to overly detail this, but this is as cathartic as talking to a friend. I have no dear friends, however, who have gone through this, so this is a very meaningful expression to me. This complete hysterectomy has been physically and emotionally devastating, not to mention, very financially taxing. My ONLY consolation is that it possibly "saved my life," but I will never know if it was absolutely, positively necessary. I know that this entire medical chain of events I went through was NOT necessary—I am sharing my story in the hopes that it will help other women take note of possible long-term consequences of traditional, and often automatic medical practices, and avoid ending up in a painful, powerless place, submitting to an enormous sacrifice in order to survive.

Thank you for the opportunity to share my story, I would like to spare any more women from the experience that I had to submit to.

—Grace - Maine USA

Writer's Profile

ଔଔଔଔଔଔଔଔଔଔଔ   ଅଅଅଅଅଅଅଅଅଅଅ

Authored by: L. Enid Miranda
Age: 58
From: Rincon, Puerto Rico

Hysterectomy: 1995
Age at surgery   50

2 Ovaries removed   1995
Age at surgery   50

Reason for
    surgery/surgeries: Fibroids and heavy periods

Hormone replacement
    history: None, I exercise, lift weights,
                        meditate, take vitamins, and eat
                        right

Other medications: Not reported

I had a hysterectomy at the age of 50 because of fibroids. My periods were so heavy, I was anemic. It was the worst decision I have ever made in my life.

Apparently, I have developed adhesions from the operation, and now after I have sex, my abdomen gets swollen and I feel a discomfort (dull ache) for about 24 hours.[2] This completely ruined my sex life! I never would have had the operation if the doctor (a woman) had told me of this possibility, but all she said was, "You don't need your uterus anymore."

Its too late for me, but I hope this will help other women make the right decision.

—L. Enid Miranda - Rincon, Puerto Rico

Writer's Profile

Authored by: Elizabeth
Age: 43
From: United Kingdom

Hysterectomy: 2000
Age at surgery   40

2 Ovaries removed   2000
Age at surgery   40

Reason for
    surgery/surgeries: Endometriosis and fibroids

Hormone replacement
    history: 2000 to present
                        Estradiol and testosterone
                        pellets

Other medications: Not reported

I have had very little opportunity to discuss my feelings with anyone. We seem to live in a society where this dreadful operation is so acceptable to so many, that it is virtually impossible to swim against the tide if you feel, as I always have, that hysterectomy and/or oophorectomy are terribly inhumane procedures.

I had one pregnancy that miscarried in the 3rd/4th month. Six months later, the abdominal pain started. I knew instinctively from the outset that this pain would stop me from having children. I went from doctor to doctor, becoming more and more desperate as they found nothing. I was diagnosed with arthritis and/or irritable bowel syndrome. The pain was crippling for two weeks in every four. I was self-employed and spending one week a month in bed. I sometimes kept my neighbours awake, screaming through the night. Often I could only urinate by sitting in a scalding hot bath, bowel movements were impossible for weeks at a time. I waited six months to see a specialist. When he diagnosed severe endometriosis, I went onto an "emergency waiting list" and I waited five more months for a laparoscopy. Moments after I woke up from the procedure, the consultant came and told me that the endometriosis and fibroid was so severe that a radical hysterectomy was the only answer. I was glad to finally know what was wrong, after having been branded a "malingerer" for seven years. A month later, I persuaded the doctor to treat me with drug therapy (100 mg Provera every day for 18 months). The side effects were terrible, but the pain was slightly relieved. I couldn't stand up straight and sex drive on Provera is zero.

A year later, I asked the doctor to refer me for laser surgery. She did, but I had to wait nine months to see the only available specialist in this area. He examined me, then told me that it was serious and said I would go on another emergency list for another laparoscopy. I then had to wait six more months. Immediately after this procedure, he told me that he could laser the endometriosis and remove the fibroid. I had to wait another three months to see him again, on which occasion he dashed all my hopes by telling me that he would never consider performing laser therapy on such bad endometriosis, and the fibroid could not be removed by any doctor. I was in serious pain all the time. I asked him about the possibility of saving anything—my cervix, ovaries, etc. He was quite brutal about the necessity to remove everything, and told me it was rubbish that my sex life would be ruined—sex in fact would be "one million times better" afterwards, although my sex drive "might be" affected. He said there was a lot of rubbish written in the press about the subject.

At the end of the ten month wait for a hospital bed, I was unable to stand for more than half an hour. I had frequent "fevers," which I attributed to a developing peritonitis, and was unable to sleep in any position in bed. However, I still had to wait another six months due to a bed shortage.

When I finally had surgery, I nearly died from blood loss in the two days that followed. The consultant described the operation as a "nightmare." I was given Fem7 patches that didn't stick, and I developed quite severe estrogen-deficiency symptoms. I was closer to suicide then than ever before. If I hadn't had my dog to care for, I would gladly have made an exit.

I now realize I can never look at a man again and feel a "stirring" in my belly, because there is nothing left to stir.[2] Recently, I've thought a lot about sex drive and what it is. It is like a language that enables you to communicate and function in society. It gives you a place and a stake in society, because you are someone who possesses something that everyone in society recognizes and values. After this operation, you find you have been struck deaf and dumb, unable to communicate or respond in any way, with your body or your emotions. Meeting an attractive man after this operation is like a wheelchair user watching a game of football. He might fantasize about playing, but the message from his brain will never reach his legs, and soon he stops fantasizing, because it is too tortuous. I feel like an outcast, a subhuman, who has no further place in society. I don't even have the justification of children. I feel disabled, ashamed of what I have become and completely useless. What I wanted to tell my consultant, but couldn't because he wouldn't let me, was that making the decision to have this operation was like deciding to turn off the life support system on the person I loved most, while at the same time, being the person attached to the life support who didn't want it switched off. It was a moral dilemma, similar to considering an abortion, it was saying good-bye to the person I once was and loved, it was consenting to the killing of the only good part of myself, it was life-denying and immoral in every respect.

The grief of having lost the dream of children is so overwhelming that I can hardly bear it. I have terrible nightmares at night. The worst one is when I dream of being the person I once was.

Personally, I want to see this operation outlawed, performed only in cases where special dispensation has been granted by a court of law to treat malignant (cancerous) conditions. I know if I had been a man all those years ago exhibiting symptoms that might had resulted in castration, no effort would have been spared to find and treat the cause of the pain. I would not have been left for seven years with only a referral to a psychiatrist. As long as this operation exists as an easy and acceptable option, no effort will be made to research, treat, or cure nonmalignant (noncancerous) conditions, which affect so many women, with alternatives that preserve the integrity of the uterus and ovaries. If these conditions, for which surgery is so often the only answer offered to women, existed in men, they would have been dealt with as a priority years ago. Women do not help their own cause by propagating this myth that it "is the best thing they ever did." I'm sure this is just false bravado so they don't have to admit what has really been done to them. If this was the best thing they ever did, what did they spend the rest of their lives doing?

—Elizabeth - United Kingdom

Writer's Profile

ఴఴఴఴఴఴఴఴఴఴఴ ಜ಼ಜ಼ಜ಼ಜ಼ಜ಼ಜ಼ಜ಼ಜ಼ಜ಼ಜ಼

Authored by: Renee Rehfeld
Age: 52
From: USA

Hysterectomy: 2002
Age at surgery   52

2 Ovaries removed   2002
Age at surgery   52

Reason for
     surgery/surgeries: Fibroids and solid mass on one
ovary

Hormone replacement
     history: 2002 to present
Tri-est and progesterone
cream, DHEA, GABA

Other medications: None

I am 51 years old. At the end of August 2002, I had a complete hysterectomy—everything gone—uterus, cervix, fallopian tubes, and ovaries, etc. It has been quite a nightmare ever since. I am sharing my story because it is pretty unbelievable. I feel off most of the time now. I also feel as though I am fighting for my life, and at the mercy of every doctor there ever was.

I had fibroids and a benign tumor on one of my ovaries. They could not tell if the tumor was benign, because it was solid in nature, so an oncologist was present and performed the actual surgery.

Three weeks after surgery, I began to feel weird. I was taking 1 mg of estradiol per day. My gynecologist increased my estradiol, but it did not seem to help. She tried Zoloft, which I also did not like. I was beginning to feel anxious, so since I had successfully taken Xanax in the past, she prescribed that as well. About three weeks later, I began having really bad anxiety, and I ended up in a hospital for 11 days where they put me on Paxil, Depakote, and Ambien. While I was in the hospital, one the doctors gave me her card and said that she believed I should see her own personal doctor. Intuitively, I felt all of the medicine they had put me on was wrong. Throughout all of this time, I kept telling everyone about my surgery, and that my problems were the result of the hormonal changes that occurred after my hysterectomy, but they did not want to listen and just put me on an estrogen patch.

When I got out of the hospital, I went to see a new doctor and she sent me to another psychologist. He finally said all of this was nonsense and sent me to see an endocrinologist, because he believed all my problems were hormonal. When I saw the endocrinologist, I tested positive for the antibodies for Graves Disease, which was brought on by the surgery. She said my thyroid was normal, however it could still cause my symptoms of anxiety. She put me on Toprol, a beta-blocker, and trazodone (another antidepressant to be taken at night for sleep).[8] However, in order for me to take the new drugs, they then had to first wean me off all of the other drugs, which was a nightmare. The Toprol is now making me lose my hair, so now I am back to: "what do I do?"

So, I decided to call my gynecologist from another state, who had taken care of me for six years. She said that I should take tri-est (estradiol, estrone, and estriol), and progesterone cream. She put me in touch with a compounding pharmacist who specializes in women's problems such as mine. He has walked me through taking the tri-est, and progesterone cream, along with taking Drenamin, Gaba, and DHEA. I am now off ALL this medication, and just on non-oral hormones, and am now beginning to feel so much better. My memory is back and I feel like I can think again. I am doing everything possible to get well, exercising every day for two hours, taking supplements three times a day, acupuncture, and eating right.

I feel like so many conventional doctors are not educated in hormone replacement therapy. They think that if we all just take an estrogen pill, we will be fine, and if we are not, they wash their hands of us and send us on our way down a very unpleasant path. Doctors' ignorance is at our expense. They really make you feel ridiculous for even trying other methods, or they really scare you into thinking that their way is the only the only way that will work. It takes courage to try other methods, especially when you are soooo sick!

After surgery, I felt like I was in a living nightmare that just would not end. Before my surgery, I was a happy young woman. My husband is a successful producer in the film business, we have two beautiful children, two homes, a good life. After surgery, I felt like I was slowly deteriorating. I was determined not to give up, but I have to say, it has been one journey I could have done without. I urge all women to educate themselves before going down this road, and don't be afraid to try other forms of HRT. I know that synthetic estrogen did not work for my body, as I am sure that I did not absorb any of it. I am grateful that I had the courage to try a non-oral route of hormone therapy—it truly is saving my life. It is a job to balance your hormones, but well worth the effort.

—Renee Rehfeld - USA

Writer's Profile

CRCRCRCRCRCRCRCRCRCR   ଅଅଅଅଅଅଅଅଅଅଅ

Authored by:	Bannon T., M.A.
Age:	49
From:	Seattle, Washington USA
Hysterectomy:	2000
Age at surgery	46
2 Ovaries removed	2000
Age at surgery	46
Reason for surgery/surgeries:	Fibroid, endometriosis, ovarian cysts, and chronic pain
Hormone replacement history:	Estratest® and Premarin® cream
Other medications:	Not reported

I am three years post-op and had a TAH/BSO. I elected to have my surgery with a local anesthetic as an outpatient procedure. I wanted to watch! I gave birth to 3 children and I really wanted to "see" the place where they all lived and grew.

My surgical team was very supportive and talked to me throughout the procedure, letting me know every step along the way. They answered my questions about their terminology when they were telling me what the sensations were that I was feeling.

One of the most surprising things to me was actually seeing my uterus and ovaries. I had only seen textbook photos and drawings before this. I was shocked to see how very small and delicate they were!

I liked being conscious throughout the procedure and got to hear them as they discovered a previously unknown severe case of endometriosis and numerous "chocolate cysts" on my ovaries. Previously I had no explanation for all the menstrual pain I'd suffered for many years. I felt relieved and vindicated in an odd way.

I had a grapefruit sized fibroid in the wall of my uterus that had been pressing against a nerve in my lower back causing severe lower back pain for several years (for which I had several courses of unsuccessful physical therapy).

One of the complications was the emergence of continual, significant, burning bladder pain that intensified for weeks and months after the surgery. I did not have an infection of any kind and went through numerous urologic tests, including a cystoscopy where they inflated the bladder to look for interstitial cystitis. Additionally, they did kidney function tests (IVP pyelogram) and found nothing. My general practitioner and urologist had no idea what to do—he did say he ran into this with postmenopausal women but didn't know why.

It wasn't until months later I went to my ob-gyn and she said, "Oh, it is lack of estrogen in your bladder! Very common."

I had been taking oral estrogen and she prescribed a small amount of vaginal estrogen cream. It took care of the problem within a week. Now, I occasionally have a recurrence of the pain, and I am able to relieve it with a few small doses of the vaginal cream.

—Bannon T., M.A. - Seattle, Washington USA

Writer's Profile

CRCRCRCRCRCRCRCRCRCR SOSOSOSOSOSOSOSOSOSO

Authored by:	Judith Isaac
Age:	61
From:	USA
Hysterectomy:	1996
Age at surgery	54
2 Ovaries removed	1996
Age at surgery	54
Reason for surgery/surgeries:	Large fibroids
Hormone replacement history:	Not reported
Other medications:	Not reported

UTERUS, FAREWELL

GOOD-BYE UTERUS
who made me a woman at age fourteen.

GOOD-BYE UTERUS
who bled with the cycles of the moon.

GOOD-BYE UTERUS
who gave rhythm and mood to my days.

GOOD-BYE UTERUS
who gave me physical pleasure.

GOOD-BYE UTERUS
who created dreams and fantasies.

GOOD-BYE UTERUS
who made me feel full and whole.

GOOD-BYE UTERUS
IN WHICH MY SON LIVED AND DIED.

UTERUS
I forgive those who took you from me.

UTERUS
I let go of you with ambivalence, pain, and love.

UTERUS
I return you to God and eternity.

—Judith Isaac

ANNIVERSARY THOUGHTS

February 22, 1996
I thought
I would die.

Instead
the surgeon only
cut out
my uterus,
my ovaries.

ONLY!

Did he also steal
my joyous laughter
my energetic step
my concentration
my sensuality?

Did he accidently
nick my soul?

—Judith Isaac
February 22, 1998

UNDERCURRENTS

On the anniversary
of the surgery
I wear
a mask of normalcy
to hide from myself,
the world
the losses

the loss
of wellness
of energy
of appetite.

When a part
is cut
from the whole,
the whole changes.
The body hurts.
The soul aches.

In this high-tech
fast-paced world
of Internet
faxes and
beepers

a woman's cry
is a whisper.

Humanity distracted,
afraid . . .
Truth is postponed.

—Judith Isaac
February 22, 1999
(3rd anniversary)

UNTITLED

Reflections, shadows
are what you see.
This dancing picture
is not me.

Teacher, poet
daughter, wife
are only the outlines
of a life.

Color in the body,
make it whole.
Alas, these pieces
are not the soul!

Are you confused?
So am I.
The question continues
to be why.

A complex being
is it's own . . . .
Only in God's eye
is it known.

—Judith Isaac
January, 2000

Writer's Profile

രുരുരുരുരുരുരുരുരുരു   ഇരുഇരുഇരുഇരുഇരുഇരു

Authored by: Della Cruse
Age: 70
From: Conroe, Texas USA

Hysterectomy: 1971
Age at surgery   38

1 Ovary removed   1971
Age at surgery   38

1 Ovary removed   1972
Age at surgery   39

Reason for
   surgery/surgeries: 1971 Cyst on ovary
                      1972 Cyst on ovary

Hormone replacement
   history: 1971 to 1997

                      1997 to present
                      Tri-est

Other medications: Not reported

I am 69 years old. At age 38, I had the surgery because of terrible problems with an ovary that kept swelling to the size of a cantaloupe. My uterus and one ovary were removed. However, 12 months later, I was in for emergency surgery to remove the other ovary.

I tried all kinds of hormone replacement therapies before one seemed to work. I had terrible depression, and contemplated suicide, but had three little children to care for, and my doctor helped me through that. I wanted to leave my husband, but didn't. I was a soprano who sang all the time. My voice completely changed, and I have lost my identity there.

By the time I was 54, I could not dress myself as a result of rheumatoid arthritis, my husband left, more depression,[9] and lots of illness.

I switched to better nutrition, natural estrogen, and used the femirone creams for several years. I am now very healthy, very happy, and just thank God that I got through all that stuff.

I have always counseled women who just had hysterectomies to mark their calendars, because in about six months they would be very unhappy with their marriage and needed to prepare themselves.

—Della Cruse - Conroe, Texas USA

Questions to Ask

Questions to ask if you are being offered prophylactic ovary removal (no cancer, only as protection from possible cancer or to avoid future surgery in the event of problems with the remaining ovary):

1. What is my actual lifetime risk of developing ovarian cancer?
2. Can I still develop ovarian cancer even after my ovaries are removed?
3. What other systems in my body are dependent on my ovarian hormones?
4. Do my ovaries really stop functioning at menopause, or do they continue producing testosterone?
5. Does loss of the ovaries and their hormones contribute to an increased risk of heart disease?
6. Does loss of the ovaries and their hormones contribute to an increased risk of osteoporosis?
7. Since teeth are bone, will I risk problems with my teeth, or loss of them, if I start losing bone due to loss of my hormones?
8. Will loss of my ovarian hormones influence my body's metabolism and lead to a possible change in my weight, either gain or loss that I cannot control?
9. Do my ovarian hormones affect my insulin sensitivity, especially if I have diabetes in my family background? Does it put me at increased risk of developing non-insulin-dependent diabetes mellitus (NIDDM)?
10. Will my thyroid keep functioning normally?

11. Is there a possibility I won't feel like myself afterwards, or undergo personality changes?

12. Will I continue to be able to be around people and enjoy being with them, as well as still emotionally connect with those I love?

13. Do all women absorb hormones the same, or do some women have trouble absorbing what is offered?

14. Is it true that hormone replacement is a trial-and-error process, which can take years to determine the correct dosage and method of delivery that can be absorbed, and some women never find hormone replacement that works well for them after surgery?

15. Can loss of estrogen cause dry skin, including dry eyes, or vaginal tissue that could make sexual activity difficult?

16. Do I face potential hair loss as a result of hormone imbalance?

17. Will my short-term memory be the same?

18. Will my brain function be the same, or can I develop mental confusion or "brain fog."

19. Will my quality of sleep and the ability to sleep soundly throughout the night be affected?

20. What is the risk of developing osteoarthritis when I lose my ovarian hormones?

21. Can I develop fibromyalgia or chronic fatigue syndrome as a result of just the surgical procedure, and then have an even higher risk due to the loss of my ovarian hormones?

Personal Notes

Family Experiences

ෲෲෲෲෲෲෲෲෲෲෲ ෨෨෨෨෨෨෨෨෨෨෨

Writer's Profile

ଔଔଔଔଔଔଔଔଔଔଔ ଔଔଔଔଔଔଔଔଔଔ

Authored by:	Peter (husband)
Age:	45
From:	Santa Monica, California USA

Wife's history:
Age:	45

Hysterectomy:	2001
Age at surgery	44

2 Ovaries removed	2001
Age at surgery	44

Reason for surgery/surgeries:	Fibroids

Hormone replacement history:	2001 to present Estrogen patch

Other medications:	None

My wife is 45 years old. At age of 44, she suffered from fibroids and was advised to have an urgent hysterectomy. She was told that she should also have her ovaries and cervix removed in order to avoid the risk of cancer later on in life.

Immediately after the operation she was given hormone patches, which was a standard low dosage without regard to her previous hormone levels, and with no planned follow-up. My wife's recovery was slow, and she was discharged from the hospital after one week.

Several months later she told me that she had been thinking and had decided she no longer loved me and wanted to leave. She also said she did not feel safe with me and did not want to be alone with me! This was confusing to me since throughout our marriage I had never given her any reason to mistrust me. When we had recently tried to have sex for the first time since her surgery, it became a frustrating experience for both of us, rather than the fulfilling enjoyment we were used to (plus it made me feel very inadequate). I don't know how much the disappointment in our sex played a role in her decision. She was obviously going through a tremendous change, which was precipitating this crisis.

I am a health professional and I work with depressed people, so I well recognized her classic depressive symptoms.[9] Obviously, however, I could not treat my wife, so I asked her to see her doctor about possible depression and to have her hormone dosage reviewed. Her doctor (a female) said that my wife's estrogen dosage had nothing to do with depression, and that her lack of physical symptoms suggested that the dosage was correct. Additionally, she stated, if my wife thought she was depressed, she should buy a book on depression, read it, and if she thought she was really depressed, then she would see her for depression!

My aim was to support my wife through what I recognized as an emotional illness, so we agreed to separate, but not divorce. Our relationship has been amicable, and there is some hope that at a point in the future we will review what has happened and perhaps get together again.

Recently, when I noticed that she had dark hair on her upper lip, downy hairs on the sides of her face and neck, and that her body shape had changed dramatically, I urged her again to see the doctor and ask about these changes. As a result, the doctor did change her hormone patch dosage and type, but my wife is still suffered from huge mood swings. I further encouraged her to see either a gynecologist or an endocrinologist, but so far she has refused, which I feel also reflects her current mental state. Her existing doctor told her she would not review how the new hormone patches were working for two months!

For me personally, I have found the last six months extremely depressing and devastating as our lives have been turned upside down. The hysterectomy was "sold" to my wife as the best thing she could do and that everything would be fine afterwards. Nobody told her about possible emotional side effects. Nobody explained what my role should or would be in supporting her. I have done everything I know to respond in a positive and supportive manner, but I am not sure anything would have helped. Certainly a less than supportive role would have lead to total destruction of any future we might have together. I just hope my support will result in our staying together, because I still love her very much.

There should be a lobby to provide much better care for all the people who are impacted by such a destructive and life-changing operation. A much broader range of information should be made available to everyone involved, including family members. I feel that the medical industry is more interested in avoiding criticism rather than in telling the truth. If we compare the information and involvement offered to new parents before, during, and after childbirth with the total "nothingness" of available information on hysterectomies, we will see that there is a great void of accurate information for women and their families. I am extremely sad that my life, my wife's, and our children have been irrevocably hurt by what has happened to her mental stability. I can only hope that by sharing my story it will help to serve as an example for others to see how these surgeries can impact a family forever. It may be too late for our family—but it is not to late for others who will hopefully find this book.

—Peter (husband) - Santa Monica, California USA

Writer's Profile

Authored by: Helen Gray (daughter)
Age: 34
From: La Mesa, California USA

Mother's history:
Age: 60
From: Sheffield England

Hysterectomy: 1987
Age at surgery   44

2 Ovaries removed   1987
Age at surgery   44

Reason for
    surgery/surgeries: Numerous benign fibroid
                         tumors

Hormone replacement
    history: None

Other medications: None

Mum's aren't supposed to get sick—ever! Who else is there to cook dinners, clean your clothes, and be there for you when you've had a bad day at school? Dads certainly aren't.

My mum had been complaining that she could feel something in her lower abdominal area—a lump or something. My mum's from the old school that doesn't complain about their health, ignores all symptoms, does the ostrich with the head stuck in the sand deal, and pretends whatever "it" is will go away. Add to the fact that being British, stiff upper lip and all, and that she is one of 11 children, nobody tolerated sickness, especially her mother.

Suffice to say it was a nightmare getting her to make an appointment to see an ob-gyn. She hadn't seen a doctor since her last child, my younger brother, born when I was 10 years old. I was now 18. So for eight years she hadn't had a pap smear or any exam. She finally made the appointment for 8:30 AM December 20. At 9:00 AM I was ushered into the headmasters office to be informed that my mother was undergoing emergency surgery to remove a seven-pound tumor. I was scared and worried. That's the size of a baby! My brother had weighed 7 pound and two ounces when he was born, only two ounces more than the tumor currently residing in her womb!

The next few days were a blur. Mum was, and still is a full-time businesswoman, and had not had time for the food shopping for Christmas. It was up to me to buy and cook the turkey and all the trimmings for Christmas dinner. It was always a very traditional and proper celebration in my household. I think my mum is Martha Stewart's twin (a well-kept secret). I had a lot to live up to, but it was the prospect of mum not being home for Christmas that was the worst fear. It just wouldn't be Christmas without her.

Thankfully, she came home on Christmas Eve, and I'll never forget how she looked. She looked as if she had aged overnight. She was stooped over as she was in pain with the stitches and had lost a lot of weight. She was slim before, but now her legs resembled match sticks. Her pallor was gray, and pain was etched in her face. I was simply relieved to have her home and safe. The tumor was benign and so were the numerous fibroids that were also found in her womb. They removed both ovaries, but left the womb intact. Why? She was offered HRT, but my mum doesn't even like to take aspirin when she has a headache and she had read reports that HRT caused breast cancer, a disease that eventually took her best friend's life. Needless to say, instead of taking the six weeks off, which the doctor had recommended, she went back to work after two weeks, being self-employed will do that to you.

She swears she has never been the same since. After a lifetime of being slightly underweight, she was now overweight, not eating any differently. She just felt that her system was "out of whack," an English term for things not being right. She became temperamental and quick to temper, after being the most tolerant and patient human being I had ever met.

Even though she has never felt the same, she has never returned for a checkup. The distrust of the NHS (National Health System in England) is probably responsible for more illness rather than healing people, due to their fear of the system.

I encourage her to go to a doctor every time I talk to her, and every week I get the same response, "maybe someday." I, on the other hand, rush to the doctor at the first sign of anything, probably the result of my mother's marked fear of them, I want to believe they can and will cure whatever ails me.

How did this affect my brothers? It didn't. The male species of our family did not seem to notice mum's behavior or moods so long as they got fed and had clean clothes. My father on the other hand got to hear about the aches and pains every day, but he is also of the same frame of mind that it's "all in the mind."

Now my mum's anguish continues as she's going through menopause. The hot flashes, more weight gain, irritable moods, depression—the list goes on. I know that whatever my future holds, the key to good health is informing yourself as to the options available to treat your condition. I wish my mum could have read a book like this book 16 years ago. Maybe she would have chosen a different path.

—Helen Gray (daughter) - La Mesa, California USA

Personal Notes

Tubal Ligation Experiences

Writer's Profile

 CBCBCBCBCBCBCBCBCBCB   🍒   ꏍꏍꏍꏍꏍꏍꏍꏍꏍꏍ

Authored by:	Maureen Parniani
Age:	39
From:	California USA
Tubal ligation:	2000
Age at surgery	36
Hysterectomy:	2002
Age at surgery	38
1 Ovary removed	2002
Age at surgery	38
Reason for surgery/surgeries:	Heavy bleeding, fibroids, and ovarian cysts
Hormone replacement history:	None
Other medications:	None

My story begins with the tubal ligation that I had in March of 2000. I was a vibrant 37 year old at the time of surgery and can pinpoint my downward slide within a few months of having this procedure done. I have been living a nightmare since.

When I was considering this procedure, I asked my ob-gyn if there would be any side effects. Would I gain weight, would my periods become heavy, etc.? He assured me nothing of the sort would happen. Having been on the pill since I was 19, I was concerned about the length of time I had been using this form of birth control method and thought this would be a safe alternative; furthermore, I had three children and was happy with the size of my family. My husband was extremely concerned about this surgery and asked my physician the same questions I had. He was assured there would be no side effects as well.

My first menstrual cycle after my surgery lasted for about a week and was very heavy. Having been on the pill I was used to very light periods lasting no more than a few days and no cramping. I was a bit surprised by this but thought this wasn't too bad considering I didn't have to worry about pregnancy anymore. Each cycle grew steadily worse. A year latter I was experiencing such horrendous periods that I would literally be bed-ridden for a few days. The cramping I experienced I could honestly compare it to the medium labor pains I felt during delivery. My sex drive was dwindling, my periods were now lasting two weeks and my PMS was horrendous. I used to think PMS was a bunch of nonsense until this. I went back to my doctor. He told me nothing was wrong and suggested I was overworked and depressed and to start taking an anti-depressant. I asked him if this had anything to do with my tubal ligation. He looked at me as if I were stupid and told me "absolutely not!" I declined the anti-depressant; I was bitchy, not depressed. I went to my internist. She put me on a medication that was supposed to help PMS symptoms. It didn't. I went to a third doctor. This doctor's office resembled a cattle-call. There were so many patients in the waiting room that people were sitting on the floor. After two hours of sitting on the floor, I was finally seen. This doctor ordered a vaginal ultrasound. This showed my uterine lining was 14 mm thick, I had a fibroid tumor as well as ovarian cysts. This physician was extremely concerned with the thickness of my uterine lining since I just finished a period that lasted 16 days three days prior! She told me I needed to have a biopsy to rule out uterine cancer. I walked out of her office devastated and scared.

The fourth doctor I went to performed a D&C in May of 2002. The results showed no signs of uterine cancer. He put me on birth control pills and told me to take two a day to see if my bleeding would slow down. It didn't. The pills gave me excruciating headaches and made me nervous. This doctor could not tell me why I was bleeding so heavy. He seemed at a loss. My next period after the D&C lasted 17 days. By now I was wearing both a tampon and pad and soaking through these within a few hours. I was also passing very large clots. My life would just about stop when my periods started. I would bleed so heavy that I would soil my clothes. Once I was standing in line at the grocery store with a full cart. I felt something on my foot (I was wearing sandals) It was blood. I rushed into the restroom. There was so much blood it looked as if someone had been murdered. Thank God I was wearing dark pants! I left the store mortified. Being the hottest part of the summer, I could no longer wear shorts, dresses, or light colored clothing. I stopped going to the gym and was afraid to take clients out or sit on anyone's furniture for fear of soiling it. In August my period lasted 47 days! I went to a 5th doctor. As I lay on his examining table I had tears streaming down my face. I was exhausted and scared. This doctor suggested two procedures: a hysterectomy or a procedure where my uterine lining was burned. The latter he said, "Would stop the bleeding, but not the pain." I was so emotionally drained and physically tired I chose the hysterectomy. I told the doctor I did not want both of my ovaries removed. We agreed on this as long as my right ovary was not diseased. I asked him about side effects. He stated, "I would feel like a new woman!" I had the surgery on September 9th. It's been a downward slide since.

After the surgery, the doctor came into my room and jubilantly told me, "I had no cancer, my uterus was enlarged and they saved my right ovary." At my 6 weeks post-op visit, the doctor did not put me on any hormone treatment and told me to enjoy my new life. I was too embarrassed to tell him I was feeling lousy. I didn't understand what I was going through. I thought I was still producing hormones because I had one ovary. It's been five months since my surgery: my sex drive is non-existent;[2] my short term memory is shot,[6] I have a hard time concentrating, I feel anxious, my gums are bleeding, I have a hard time sleeping,[8] and am depressed most of the time.[9] My PMS is still raging even though I don't have the marker of a period. I am now seeing an endocrinologist who was aghast that my doctor never followed up. I didn't even know I had endometriosis or that my cervix was removed during the surgery. I found this out not from my ob-gyn but from my endocrinologist. Did I need a hysterectomy? I don't know. I've never been told what caused my bleeding.

What happened to the pistol I used to be? The carefree, fun-loving wife and mother are gone, and in her place is someone I and my family don't recognize. It takes everything I have just to get out of bed in the morning, paste on a smile and go to work. I honestly don't know how I've kept it together. I hope the hormonal pellets I am going to have implanted will work.

—Maureen Parniani - California USA

Writer's Profile

ପ୍ରପ୍ରପ୍ରପ୍ରପ୍ରପ୍ରପ୍ରପ୍ର ಬುಬುಬುಬುಬುಬುಬುಬುಬುಬು

Authored by: Theresa Martinez
Age: 43
From: Eagan, Minnesota USA

Hysterectomy: 1996
Age at surgery   39

2 Ovaries removed   1996
Age at surgery   39

Reason for
   surgery/surgeries: Uterine fibroid and scarred
                    ovary

Hormone replacement
   history: 1996 to present
                    Premarin®, estradiol,
                    progesterone cream, birth
                    control pill, patch, and
                    Estroven®

Other medications: Not reported

I am 43 years old and the mother of four children. After my last child was born in 1993, I had my tubes tied as I was done having children. I immediately began having great menstrual problems. I began to experience pelvic pain each month, and severely heavy periods. After explaining why I have heavy periods, pelvic pain, and anemia, my gynecologist gave me several options emphasizing that after trying any of these, the ultimate cure would be a hysterectomy. He advised me to give it thought and recommended reading books that were both for and against hysterectomies. I also had ultrasounds and laparoscopy, which showed fibroid tumors, the largest one being in the uterine wall. I did read books on hysterectomy and concluded that I needed instant relief, so I scheduled a hysterectomy in July of 1996. At the time, all I can recall is being desperate for relief from the pain and the loss of blood, which left me listless. I cannot forget the extremely painful cramps that worsened after my tubal sterilization.

My doctor suspected that one of my ovaries would need to be removed since the laparoscopy showed much scar tissue on the ovary, opposite the side where I was having most of my pelvic pain. My discussion with his nurse during my pre-op visit convinced me that I did not want to have to come back years later to have my other ovary removed, like she had to after her own hysterectomy. Based on these discussions, I told the doctor, just minutes before the surgery, to remove both of my ovaries. However, the thought of estrogen replacement therapy for the remainder of my life did not occur to me and was not discussed by my doctor.

The first week following my surgery, I felt so great and optimistic that I had thought it would be a beginning of a new painless life, and that I would be able to redirect my energy to my children, and to taking care of my health. By the fourth week, however, I began to have a great deal of back pain and exhaustion just from normal grocery shopping. I still experienced pelvic pain in the same area where my ovaries were prior to the surgery.[5] I was also experiencing severe depression.[9]

At the age of 21, I was diagnosed with hyperthyroidism. Due to my trust in doctors, I asked the ears, nose, and throat specialist I was referred to which he thought was the best treatment option. Since he recommended the radioactive iodine option, that is what I chose. I was never informed that I would be on thyroid medication for the remainder of my life as a result of having this treatment. I have been taking Synthyroid for the past 20 years. Since the hysterectomy I have been reacting differently to my medication, and I have had trouble keeping my thyroid under control. I have known all along that this surgery has left me physically and mentally disabled somehow, but I have been left to feel like it is all in my head. I have not been to one doctor that has not said I have symptoms of depression and I should consider antidepressants. I resisted—I researched—I read the latest books on thyroid and estrogen. I now know that the symptoms of low thyroid mimic low estrogen, and that depression is very common after a hysterectomy. I have given up on trying to convince my doctors that I know my body and I feel that it is a physical (chemical) depression, and that I am not feeling an emotional depression. I have had the worst times of my life since I had my surgery, but I remain hopeful and optimistic of having my health restored. I allowed my doctors to persuade me to try many different antidepressants, but I have not had relief from the depression that set in after my hysterectomy. It seems worse October through April and seems to be somewhat milder during the warmer, summer-like months. In addition to battling depression, I also experience joint pain. My other new problem is that I now weigh 180, which is an extra 50 pounds on my small 5' 3" frame.[13] Before surgery, my highest weight was 155. I feel like I have been through hell since the surgery.

I should mention I also had my bladder repaired with the surgery that removed my uterus, cervix, fallopian tubes, and both ovaries. So not only did my female genitalia change, but my bladder also has never been the same. Sex and orgasms will never be as satisfying as it was before.[2]

I have been a single parent since the surgery. My kids have had to witness my horrific mood swings and severe depression. The depression feels more physical than mental. My body just seems to shut down after work each night, and by the end of the week it takes the whole weekend to recover. I am not able to function at my job like I used to, and need to, in order to support my family. I cannot lose this extra weight, as I now also do not have the energy to do so.

I have been divorced, remarried, and am in the process of a divorce from my third marriage. I experienced infidelity and abuse in my marriages. I feel as though I may have avoided these relationships had I been normal and healthy. But, I was not only weak physically, but mentally as well. It is my heart's desire to see women get healthy and have the same medical treatment as men. I have tried conjugated estrogens, estradiol and Loestrin for hormone replacement. I am still trying to find a doctor that is sincerely concerned with my health and understands what I am experiencing. I continue in my quest for restoration of my health and well-being for the sake of my younger two children who have been suffering right along with me.

—Theresa Martinez - Eagan, Minnesota USA

Writer's Profile

ෲෲෲෲෲෲෲෲෲෲෲ 🍒 ෨෨෨෨෨෨෨෨෨෨෨

Authored by: Sherry Dykes
Age: 32
From: Kingsport, Tennessee USA

Hysterectomy: 2002
Age at surgery 31

2 Ovaries removed 2002
Age at surgery 31

Reason for
    surgery/surgeries: Endometriosis

Hormone replacement
    history: 2002 to present
Prempro™

Other medications: None

I was married at 19 and like most women I wasn't ready to start a family. I chose to stay on "the pill" for four years until I was ready to become a mother. After my daughter was born in 1995, I had trouble going back on the pill. Headaches came with my cycles every month, which did not go away for a week. I was troubled with this for four years, constantly changing pill brands and doses, thinking that would fix everything.

I decided to have a tubal ligation when I couldn't stand it any longer. That went well for about six months. Then I developed an almost constant ache in my lower abdomen, which was diagnosed as endometriosis. After another diagnostic laparoscopic surgery, my ob-gyn suggested a hysterectomy. I put it off for as long as I could. There were Lupron shots for three months that drove my family away. I felt like I had no other option, but to proceed with the surgery. In May of 2002, I gave in and did what my doctor recommended. I had seen him for many years, and trusted that he knew what was best.

Six weeks after surgery and with no estrogen, I felt worse than I had ever felt in my life. So, my doctor started me on estrogen and progesterone replacement. There were many a hot flash, and a lot of torture to my family. Lashing out at my daughter for almost no reason at all was the worst. Now here I am 31 and thankful that I still have my husband by my side—no matter what. The scars are still very real and something that will never go away. I have to accept that I will have to take hormones daily, and cannot have that very important part of myself back.

When I asked my doctor if he left my cervix when he took my ovaries and uterus, he politely said, "No, you don't need it anyway." After much research, I have found out that it does have a purpose. Someone forgot to tell him that.

Since my hysterectomy I have realized that I cannot wait quite so long in between rest rooms, and making love to my husband will never be the same.

—Sherry Dykes - Kingsport, Tennessee USA

Writer's Profile

CBCBCBCBCBCBCBCBCBCB   🍏   ꙅꙅꙅꙅꙅꙅꙅꙅꙅꙅ

Authored by: Dawn
Age: 40
From: Sanford, Florida USA

Hysterectomy: 2001
Age at surgery   38

1 Ovary removed   2001
Age at surgery   38

1 Ovary removed   2002
Age at surgery   39

Reason for
    surgery/surgeries: Adenomyosis, fibroids, cysts,
                        heavy bleeding, and painful
                        intercourse

Hormone replacement
    history: 2002 to present
                        Estratest FS®, Cenestin®
                        (conjugated estrogens), and
                        Estrace® (estradiol)

Other medications: Not reported

I went to my primary care doctor complaining of heavy periods, severe cramping, painful intercourse, and severe PMS. I was given a referral for an ultrasound within the week. It was discovered that I had some really large fibroids on and in my uterus. I was then given a referral to an ob-gyn. He in turn ordered another ultrasound, which showed the fibroids growing. At my next appointment, he recommended a hysterectomy. He told me that since my tubes had already been tied, and I no longer had the desire to have children, this was the best thing. He would take the uterus and cervix, and try to save one of my ovaries. I got the impression I had no other choice and that my condition was detrimental to my health. I had my hysterectomy on August 30, 2001. I was given a bikini cut following the scar that ran from four previous C-sections. I was told I had numerous cysts and fibroids that were "eating your uterus," adenomyosis, and major adhesions. He said he was able to save the left ovary, as it appeared healthy.

At two weeks post-op, I went to have my staples removed, and complained of pain in the left lower pelvic area. I was told this was normal healing and would go away. At three weeks, I went back for fever, pain, and a general "I'm not doing any better" feeling. Again, I was told this was normal healing and to give it time. By the time I was five weeks post-op, I was complaining of major pain again, bleeding, pain on urination, and fever. I was told I had a urinary tract infection and was ordered a prescription for the pharmacy. I took the antibiotic for a week and had no relief. My fever was going up to 101-102 at times. I was vomiting and bleeding. I was told I was having an allergic reaction to the antibiotic and to stop taking it. I went back to the doctor at eight weeks post-op, and had not had any improvement at all. My doctor finally did a pelvic exam again and said I may have vaginal cuff cellulitis (inflammation of surgical wound) and wanted me admitted to the hospital ASAP. It took another seven days and fever spikes up to 103-105 for them to do a CAT scan. I ended up in the hospital for ten days. It turned out I had numerous abscesses on my cuff, and cysts on my remaining ovary. I was given a percutaneous drain and mega doses of antibiotics, and I did feel better after this was done. I asked my emergency room surgeon about the cyst on my remaining ovary and was told, "well, maybe it will burst on its own."

I went home and tried to heal. For a few weeks, I did feel better than I had since having the surgery. I continued having pain in my left side and went back to my surgeon. Again, I was told things were normal although I now had a small hernia near my belly button. My surgeon released me from his care and told me to go back to my primary doctor for any future problems. It would take the next six months to convince doctors that something still wasn't right. When I went back to the primary doctor, I was referred to another ob-gyn. I was refused an appointment as I was still less than six months from my previous surgery, and was told to go back to the original surgeon. This time I refused, as I was just not comfortable with someone that refused to believe my pain. I finally ended up on the phone with a nurse in tears begging her to get me in to a doctor that would at least check things out for me. When I did get in to see my primary care doctor and explained to him what I had been going through, he did a pelvic exam. What he found was incredible to him—let alone me. I had severe granulation on my cuff. I had a hole in my cuff that had either come apart or never been sewn properly to begin with. Through this hole I had a prolapsed fallopian tube. I had another abscess on my cuff that had become infected also. He told me this was "surgery related," and I needed to see my surgeon as soon as possible.

I went BACK to the surgeon and was reprimanded for not coming to him sooner. I told him I tried to, and was told it was normal healing. Again, I was sent back to surgery in April of 2002, which led to another six weeks of initial healing. This time

I had adhesions lysed, my left ovary and tube removed, along with the cysts and abscesses that had attached to it, as well as repair of the vaginal cuff. However, he did NOT fix the hernia while he was in there. Again, I was sent home. Exactly two weeks later I complained of pain in my left side, and again I was told it was normal healing. "I did a lot of work and you will feel it for awhile," is what I was told. He put me on hormone replacement therapy and told me to come back in four weeks. Again, I had to fight for another seven months to find the cause of my pain. At one point I was told, "It's impossible for you to feel pain as you have nothing left." I was never checked. I was never tested. I let it go hoping that he was right. Then, I was referred by my primary physician to a general surgeon for my hernia, but I could not find one to fix it due to the pelvic pain I was still having.[5] Also, they did not feel I was healthy enough to undergo surgery again so soon.

In October of 2002, I finally ended up in the emergency room due to severe pain in my left side. The pain was so bad that I could not stand-up. I was given an ultrasound, and it was discovered that I had a "prominent left ovary with cysts." The surgeon that performed my hysterectomy was called and the emergency room doctor was told by my surgeon, "That's impossible . . . she just has adhesions. Send her home and tell her to make an appointment with my office." The ER doctor threw up his hands and said, "There is nothing more I can do. Come back if the pain gets worse." I made an appointment with the head doctor at my surgeon's practice, and spoke with him. The CT scan came back with the same results, "prominent left ovary." I was not given the option of another appointment with him as his nurse called and referred me to a gyn-oncologist. Her words were, "This is out of his league and he doesn't know what to do." Again, I was given another CT scan. Again, the same results! While waiting for the results, as I was walking from my bath to the living room I had the worst pain I could ever imagine. The pain was so bad it sent me to my knees and I was sick for the next three days. I went back to the oncologist and was given another ultrasound to see if the cyst had grown. It hadn't. It had burst and that was the pain I had felt. I still had a 5 cm "mass" on the left side that "could be" an ovary or an ovarian remnant. It had to be removed.

This past November 2002 I had surgery one more time to remove this "ovary." I had to have a vertical cut this time as I had had too many surgeries in the past, and she felt I would heal better with a new incision. She fixed my hernia this time, which was the size of a golf ball. The pathology report showed:

> lyses of adhesions, removal of left pelvic mass, removal of several cysts, removal of an abscessed stitch from the last surgery.

My adhesions were tremendous again this time. My oncologist had to separate my bowels, my ureter, and my cuff from all that they were adhered to. On trying to remove the "mass', it burst before it could make it to pathology as a whole. It showed in the report it was ovarian in nature but until it is investigated further we will not know if it was a whole or a remnant. This time my oncologist used a barrier called intercede to help avoid future adhesions. I again experienced immediate surgical menopause, and had to increase my estrogen due to the fact that I finally had no ovary producing hormones.

It is now January 2003, and I am nine weeks post-op from, this, my third abdominal surgery. I feel like I am finally healing. I am growing stronger everyday, and finally for the first time in the 17 months since my original hysterectomy, I have no internal pain. I am weak from having so many surgeries in such a short amount of time but know that this will get better. It has been a hard long road to "fight" for my own health care. There were many times I wanted to give up, but thanks to a wonderful group of ladies I call my "sisters" from a hysterectomy support Website, I came through. I am stronger mentally and emotionally. I will never be the woman I was before my hysterectomy, but I think I like this new me now. Do I regret having the hysterectomy? Not at all. I regret that doctors don't listen to their patients when they say they are in pain. I regret that doctors have forgotten that women DO know their own bodies. I regret that doctors treat people as numbers and go for the almighty dollar. We go to them for help and they have convinced themselves that everyone is the same. There doesn't seem to be room for the person who may be healing or feeling things differently. I wish I had known and researched so much more before I agreed to my hysterectomy—alternatives . . . treatments . . . outcomes . . . risks. Knowledge is power. And sometimes you have to just fight for that knowledge for your own well-being.

I travel a new road now . . . one to a better me that I am comfortable and happy with. I have come to realize the little things don't matter. What I went through has not only affected myself, but my 17 year old daughter and the wonderful man who stuck with me through all of this. I haven't been able to work for almost two years now. It will take some time to put things in my personal life back together, as I have focused so long on just my health. This time . . . I will have my life back.

—Dawn - Sanford, Florida USA

Questions to Ask

Questions to ask if you are deciding on a tubal ligation for birth control:

1. Will I continue having normal menstrual cycles?

2. Will my periods change in frequency or flow?

3. Is there a possibility of my ovarian function being hampered in any way?

4. Do women have a greater frequency of ovarian cysts after a tubal?

5. Do women have a greater frequency of fibroid tumors after a tubal?

6. What percentage of women who have a tubal need a hysterectomy later?

7. Is this percentage greater than that in the normal population who have not have a tubal ligation?

Resolution
Without
Surgery

ഌഌഌഌഌഌഌഌഌഌഌഌ ജ്ജ്ജ്ജ്ജ്ജ്ജ്ജ്ജ്ജ്ജ്

Writer's Profile

Authored by: Glenda Tall
Age: 67
From: Boston, Massachusetts USA

Hysterectomy: No
Age at surgery   N/A

Ovaries removed   No
Age at surgery   N/A

Reason for
    surgery/surgeries: N/A

Hormone replacement
    history: 1989 to 2000

Other medications: Not reported

In the 1970s, as a young mother of three sons, I began to suffer severe pain in my lower abdomen. It was seemingly unrelated to menstruation, although the pre-menstrual days of each month were even worse. My stomach was distended and hard. The pain was such that involuntary tears became common. My gynecologist told me that the problem was endometriosis and that he would recommend a hysterectomy. I repeatedly asked if there was any other treatment that would help, but he insisted I should agree to the hysterectomy. I chose not to.

In the late 1970s, I was treated with a Chinese herbal formula in capsule form. Within three months, the pain was greatly diminished, and soon thereafter, gone—forever.

At my next regular checkup, I provided my gynecologist with a packet of information regarding the treatment that had cured me, with the hope that it might help others. Years later, when he retired, the unopened packet was returned along with my medical records

—Glenda Tall - Boston, Massachusetts USA

Writer's Profile

CRCRCRCRCRCRCRCRCRCRCR   ಬುಬುಬುಬುಬುಬುಬುಬುಬುಬು

Authored by:	Donna L. Scott
Age:	43
From:	Amarillo, Texas USA
Hysterectomy:	No
Age at surgery	N/A
Ovaries removed	No
Age at surgery	N/A
Reason for surgery/surgeries:	N/A
Hormone replacement history:	None
Other medications:	None

I had two irregular periods this past summer and since it was time for my annual Pap smear, I decided to visit my gynecologist a month early. My doctor ordered a sonogram, saying that my uterus felt larger than when I was examined the year before. The sonogram showed something that was not too big in my uterus (probably fibroids, said the sonogram technician), and a cyst on one of my ovaries. In the subsequent visit to my doctor, his first statement to me was, "You need surgery." He proceeded to tell me that my uterus was "very large" and that I had "multiple fibroids." He also told me that it was up to me whether I kept my ovaries or not, but that he would like permission to remove them "if I get in there and see that they're bad." I was shocked, because in my entire adult life I've never had any gynecological problems whatsoever. I've always had regular periods, normal pregnancies, and normal Pap smears. He said the sooner we had it done the better, and for me to plan on taking a "nice six-week vacation." He scheduled the surgery for the following Wednesday, just seven days from this visit.

I went home and immediately started reading about fibroids, ovarian cysts, and hysterectomies. What I found was astonishing, and led me to believe that I certainly wasn't a candidate for a hysterectomy and possible oophorectomy. My two little irregular periods were nothing compared to the case histories I read! I also read *Your Guide to Hysterectomy, Ovary Removal, and Hormone Replacement*, which informed me of the unmentioned complications from hysterectomy and how it can turn your life upside down. I decided by the end of the weekend that I couldn't have the surgery the following Wednesday and when I phoned my doctor to inform him of my decision, he was clearly agitated and short with me. I asked him what options other than hysterectomy were available to me and he said, "None! If you don't have the surgery, you'll continue to have problems." I also asked him what kind of ovarian cyst I had and he replied, "I don't know—I can't tell until I get in there."

I went to another doctor for a second opinion a couple of weeks later. This doctor scheduled a saline sonogram, which would give a better look at my uterus and ovaries. What was found by this sonogram was that I had a polyp in the lining of my uterus, about 1 cm in size, and NO FIBROIDS. The ovarian cyst was a functional cyst (this *could* be determined from the sonogram) and would most likely dissolve on its own. The doctor also said that my uterus was NOT large for a woman who had had three pregnancies. He informed me that it is not uncommon for women in their early forties to start having irregular periods, because ovulation doesn't occur every month. He took a biopsy of the polyp to check for cancer and said there was less than a 1% chance that it would be positive (the results were negative), and he advised a D&C and removal of the polyp with a hysteroscope. That's it. I haven't had this simple procedure done yet, but my irregularities have subsided and I don't have any other symptoms. I almost had a hysterectomy for nothing! I also feel that the doctor would have taken out my ovaries based on what I have read. After all, he can't exactly tap me on the shoulder during surgery and ask me what I want him to do with them.

I hope and pray that all women facing this situation will take a little time to think, read, and seek other opinions before having any surgery done. Also, never ignore your "inner voice" when things just don't add up. We know our bodies better than anyone. I'm grateful for the information that's out there, and especially for *Your Guide to Hysterectomy, Ovary Removal, and Hormone Replacement*. It saved me from a terrible, *unnecessary* mistake.

—Donna L. Scott - Amarillo, Texas USA

Writer's Profile

Authored by:	Christine Kent
Age:	50
From:	Albuquerque, New Mexico USA
Hysterectomy:	No
Age at surgery	N/A
Ovary removed	No
Age at surgery	N/A
Reason for surgery/surgeries:	Bladder suspension in 1993 for very slight urinary incontinence, which resulted in a prolapsed uterus
Hormone replacement history:	None
Other medications:	None

Snagged by the same trap ensnaring a million women per year in the United States, I came out relatively unscathed—but still severely damaged—by the cultural phenomenon known as gynecologic surgery. During a routine pelvic examination I was diagnosed with a large uterine fibroid and bluntly advised by my gynecologist that I needed a hysterectomy. Other than occasional episodes of leaking slight amounts of urine when I coughed or sneezed I was experiencing no symptoms of pelvic difficulty whatsoever. Although it was becoming common knowledge at the time that fibroids are almost never malignant (not cancer), are extremely prevalent in the industrialized world, are diet sensitive, and stop growing at menopause, my doctor made my condition sound serious and suspicious as she urged me toward consent. I quickly sought a second opinion and was told that yes, a hysterectomy was really the only reasonable option for me.

Although my mother and sister had been hysterectomized and both tried to help me see value in the operation, my instincts told me NO WAY. I called my trusted gynecologist from years earlier when I lived in another part of the country. He assured me the fibroid could be removed by modern laser surgery and there was probably no need for hysterectomy. Relieved and resigned to the inevitable *myomectomy* (fibroid removal), within a month I was on an airplane and in the hands of my doctor, a well-educated ob-gyn who practices medicine at one of the most prestigious hospitals in California.

After examining me and inquiring of any and all symptoms I was having, I told him of my recent episodes of mild urinary incontinence. He replied that I was "too young for that kind of thing" and recommended I have my bladder "tucked up" as long as he was "going to be in there anyway." I asked him to describe any and all risks to which he responded there were none outside the usual surgical risks of anesthesia and infection, and that there might be a slight change in the stream of my urine. It all sounded safe and sensible to me. Little did I know that every part of my being had been encultured to mistrust my own judgment about the workings of my body and to trust completely in this handsome, well-established man in the white coat.

We were scheduled for surgery the following day. Believing it was a necessity, I was looking forward to it, but also felt that it was an aggravating consequence of having a female body. After the usual surgical preparation and total anesthesia, my pelvic cavity was accessed by *laparotomy* through a low incision just above the pubic bone. The fibroid, the size of a large egg, was removed using the laser, and the wound in my uterus sewn closed with permanent sutures. The "tucking up" of my bladder was accomplished via the Marshall-Marchetti-Krantz procedure—a major surgical operation where, after dissecting and tunneling down behind my pubic bone layer upon layer of skin, fat, connective tissue, nerve, lymph nodes, and blood vessels until my bladder and urethra were exposed and filled with blue dye for easier visualization. The neck of my bladder was re-angled and the connective tissue surrounding it securely sutured to the muscle of my abdominal wall. My initial recovery was "uneventful" with the associated nausea, vomiting, extreme pain and tearing sensation as I retched for hours in reaction to the anesthesia. A supra-pubic catheter (a small tube that is placed by puncturing directly through the abdominal wall and into the bladder) used to evaluate the post-surgical flow of my urine was found to have a leak in the tubing, but luckily I did not develop an infection.

When the doctor and I agreed I was strong enough to make the trip home I traveled back on the airplane with plenty of pain medication on board and abdominal dressing intact. A few weeks after the surgery I was feeling well enough to walk outside under the brilliant Indian summer sun. As I was walking back across the yard toward my house I felt an odd sensation in my vagina, rather like a tampon falling out. Not quite registering the experience, I walked slowly into the bathroom to investigate, only to encounter a large "something" bulging from my vagina. To say the least I was terrified to find an internal organ protruding from my body. In a panic, I called my California gynecologist and explained my situation. With shock and disbelief in his voice he exclaimed, "How in the world did *that* happen?" I high-tailed it to my local doctor who diagnosed it as a stage three uterine prolapse. I called the surgeon back to tell him the news and he replied that unfortunately my uterine suspension was completely unsuccessful, and this was now a truly serious condition that required hysterectomy.

I never spoke to the California physician again. Even with my rudimentary knowledge of anatomy and physiology I knew the bladder surgery had caused my uterus to prolapse. I sent for my operative report and was outraged to see the long list of risks and complications (prolapse not among them) he stated to have discussed with me. He also stated that because of my "significant incontinence, the operative procedure was *first suggested by the patient*," (which I most certainly did not).

I saw a total of four more gynecologists in an effort to gather as much information as possible about uterine prolapse. I was not interested in any more surgical "solutions" and three of the four treated me as if I were out of my mind for thinking I could manage prolapse naturally for the rest of my life. I found it amazing both male and female gynecologists had the very same conceptual framework. At best, they merely tolerated ideas and suggestions outside their area of expertise. In any event, I was fitted for a *pessary* (a rubbery diaphragm-like devise to hold up prolapsed pelvic organs) and began learning and intuiting everything I could about naturalizing my pelvic floor.

My progress was slow and discouraging at first. Parts of my pubic area near the surface scar were (and still are) completely numb. Urination now required great effort. On the lower right side deep into my pelvic cavity dwelled a constant, dull ache. My bowels behaved differently, and the glands above my pubic bone became swollen and sore with too much sexual activity. Sex itself was no longer working as it had before the surgery. Certain positions were very painful to maintain and it was as if my whole vagina had been repositioned. My menstrual periods also became very difficult. Where once menstruation was regular, relatively pain-free and unobtrusive, now each month I had to deal with pain and heaviness in my abdomen, lower back, legs, and even the arches of my feet! Most discouraging was the big, boggy uterus bulging out between my legs.

Shortly after the surgery I found a Website that is dedicated to helping women who are suffering with prolapse and similar conditions. Started by a woman who was suffering from prolapse herself, it is the only one of its kind, containing valuable information, physician referrals, and offering a forum for women. The numbers of women writing in are great, the vast majority of whom were young, healthy women in their 20s and 30s. It was through reading their postings that I began to see into the deeper nature of this widespread cultural epidemic.

The women talked amongst themselves about pessaries, exercise, "going under the knife," as well as sharing an endless array of post-surgical complications, failures, and subsequent procedures. So striking to me was how little confidence the women had in their own ability to improve their condition, and their complete faith in the urogynecologists despite the pain, limitation, damage, and exasperation continually expressed in their forum.

As I began to live well with my prolapse and to reverse my condition, I checked into the site less frequently as I witnessed it become more biased towards advocating surgery. Presently on this site, one can find the same hope, faith, and trust in the "urogynies," alongside the same tragic stories of pain, limitation, failure, and frustration.

Today my uterus is small, asymptomatic, and tucked halfway up into my vagina. At 50, I garden, run, lift heavy objects, have regular, and pain-free menstrual cycles. I do live with groin pain after an evening of vigorous dancing or a long day hike, these being my visceral "scars" from an encounter with pelvic floor surgery, as well as my "badges" for refusing to take part in a system immersed in a deep and dangerous crisis of perception.

I thank God I did not take the surgical "cure" offered to me for my prolapsed uterus. It easily could have been performed, given the vague and ambivalent consent form I unwittingly signed. Because I have all my pelvic organs, I've been able to counteract much of the damage created by the surgery. I will never be completely successful in this effort however, and will live the rest of my life fighting pain and disability from one of the hundreds of armaments waged by gynecology's war on women.

—Christine Kent - Albuquerque, New Mexico USA

Author of *Saving the Whole Woman: Natural Alternatives to Damaging "Corrective " Surgery for Pelvic Organ Prolapse and Urinary Incontinence*

Writer's Profile

ಬಬಬಬಬಬಬಬಬಬಬ ಜಜಜಜಜಜಜಜಜಜಜ

Authored by:	Anita L. Phillips
Age:	53
From:	Elmira, New York USA
Hysterectomy:	No
Age at surgery	N/A
Ovary removed	No
Age at surgery	N/A
Myomectomy:	1980s
Age at surgery	30s
Reason for surgery/surgeries:	Pain from fibroids
Hormone replacement history:	1998 to 1999
Other medications:	Not reported

I am currently 52 years old and have been experiencing all the symptoms of menopause. I have had three pregnancies. Two resulted in miscarriage, and one resulted in my 24 year old son—the joy of my life. Back in the early 80s, I had several laparoscopies and also one major uterine surgery to remove a fibroid tumor. I was trying to conceive and carry another baby successfully to term. I was seeing a fertility specialist at a large metropolitan teaching hospital, having been referred by my local gynecologist. When I reached the age of 34, I decided it was time to quit trying. I had a child and that was a blessing from God. I also made this decision because during my last "day surgery" I went into cardiac arrest and wound up staying in the hospital five days! I was advised by a team of physicians at the hospital not to have any more elective surgery, because they could not determine why this happened. However, all my previous surgeries had "complications" of one kind or another. I'm just not a good surgical candidate (for example: I had problems with anesthesia, got pneumonia, collapsed lung, etc.).

In July 1991, at age 41, I started experiencing excruciating pain at mid-month. The pain extended across my lower abdomen to the right side, down my leg to my knee. I have a high pain tolerance, but this was absolutely unbearable. It would wake me up in the middle of the night; I would become nauseous and have diarrhea. The pain would last for two weeks before every period. Motrin was all I could take because I have a stomach intolerance to pain medication. I lived on 800 mg Motrin, but it really didn't even touch the pain. Thank God I have an understanding employer, because I missed a lot of work as a result.

I went to my local gynecologist (a fellow from the old school) and he told me I probably had an ovarian cyst and his solution was, "Just keep an eye on it and let me know if it gets worse." He really wasn't listening to me—how much worse could it get!

Well, he finally retired and I found another doctor. This doctor told me that ovarian cysts usually go away in a couple of months—I had been living with this pain for about five years by this time. He told me that I had "adhesions" and suggested a complete hysterectomy. He said he would be doing an abdominal surgical procedure instead of a vaginal procedure, because he suspected the adhesions were attached to my bowel. He explained that the hormones a woman produces from mid-cycle on cause these adhesions to react and that was why I was experiencing all the pain. I told him about my poor surgical history and signed a release for him to get the information from the teaching hospital where I had my surgeries. On my next appointment, he had a typed report from the hospital and he said, "Oh, these things happen; it's just a risk you'll have to take." (I'm sitting there thinking, it's my body, my risk, my life, and my decision!) I asked him if the pain would go away when I started menopause and he said, "Yes, of course. The hormones will not be there to aggravate the adhesions." He didn't even realize it, but he had just given me the information I needed to become PROACTIVE in my own health care. I told him, "I would think about it." Fourteen months later, I started menopause. When I called the office for something else, the nurse said, "Weren't you supposed to have a hysterectomy?" My reply was, "No, I said I'd think about it; I thought about it—for about five seconds and I'm not having a hysterectomy!" I am still going through menopause and because of these adhesions I cannot take any hormone replacement therapy. I tried it all, even the natural stuff made up by a pharmacist especially for my condition, and guess what? The pain comes back worse then before. No HRT for me. So, I have been living with the hot flashes, night sweats, mood swings, etc., but I'll tell you what—IT SURE BEATS PAIN! Because I can't take the HRT, I've been loading up on my calcium, vitamin E, and soy menopause supplements (I've heard pro and con about the soy supplements).

I come from a large Italian family. My family and friends believe that the doctor is "always right," and some of them have gone like lambs to the slaughter and had hysterectomies and they still don't feel good.

I really want to tell other women out there that they need to become proactive in their own health care—read, read, read everything you can about hysterectomies, menopause, and women's health. Before you make that big decision (and, yes, you can DIE from this surgery), get a second opinion, and just to be safe; get a third if the second is the same as the first. We are not "lambs." Listen to your body, listen to your "gut feelings" and if you have a doctor who doesn't listen to YOU, dump him and find one who will.

I know some women who were young (childbearing years) when they had their hysterectomies; so, if you're a young woman, especially if you HAVE children, get all the information you can get. A hysterectomy is major surgery—it's no picnic. I almost died in "day surgery" when I went in for a laparoscopy. I had a nine-year old son at home. Who would be his "mommy" if I didn't come home? Who would read to him, who would be there at his high school and college graduations, his wedding, the birth of my grandchildren, etc.? And if you are a young woman who has not had a child yet, all the more reason to get that second, and third opinion! Think about it! Granted, we don't have medical degrees, but you're smarter than you think. READ!

I am currently a Senior Case Manager working with young mothers and I try every day to teach them to become "proactive" in their health care. They are so young and have so much to learn and I don't want them to learn the hard way!

Everybody's situation is different so that's why it's important to find out all you can about your particular condition—BEFORE you make that decision. In my case, I know I made the right one.

I hope my story will help someone out there to make the right decision. God bless and protect all of you!

—Anita L. Phillips – Elmira, New York USA

Epilogue

This collection of women's experiences distinctly shows the wide range of responses women have to these procedures. It is not clear-cut for any of them. Hysterectomy and/or ovary removal is truly a gamble. No woman knows for sure whether it will be the "best" or the "worst" thing that ever happened to her. These stories clearly reveal that the answers to the myriad problems women experience from fibroids, endometriosis, heavy perimenopausal bleeding, adenomyosis, to ovarian cysts are not as simple as removing the uterus and/or ovaries. Even when the ovaries are left in place, there is no guarantee the ovaries will remain functional, sending many women into premature menopause, with all the attending costs to their health, and ultimately to our medical system. The hormones produced by the ovaries impact every other bodily system. Without our ovarian hormones women are much more prone to heart disease, osteoporosis, depression, fibromyalgia, osteoarthritis, and cognitive brain dysfunction including memory loss, etc. Additionally, the disruption to the brain's biochemistry leads many of these women to consistently say, "I no longer feel like me!" Equally, as these stories attest, the uterus performs functions other than just childbearing. With any pelvic organ removal, there is the possibility for the remaining organs to prolapse, leading to new problems and in some instances a poorer quality of life. In far too many cases, the adhesions created by cutting into the abdominal cavity can lead to as much, or even more pain, than the conditions from which these women were seeking relief. All these potential outcomes make it clear that preservation of the uterus and ovaries is of vital importance for women's future health.

More research in the area of women's reproductive health is imperative. Some alternatives are being utilized today that do resolve women's immediate problems of bleeding and/or pain. However, when there is a disruption to the natural functions of the uterus and ovaries, such as a cutting off of the blood supply, or destruction of chemical producing cells, these alternatives can lead to new problems for the women who undergo such procedures.

With up to 1/3 of American women being hysterectomized by the age of 60, and with at least 1/3 of them experiencing tremendous problems, there are millions of women whose health has been negatively impacted. It is time for our miraculous advances in birth control, child birthing, and solutions for reproductive organ problems, which have been tremendously instrumental in reducing women's pain and suffering, to embrace the recognition that all the organs, hormones, and chemicals in the body are intricately interrelated—all working in a very delicate balance—each playing non-expendable roles in maintaining life-long vibrant health. All future research needs to develop answers that solve women's reproductive health issues in ways that honor the body's harmonious ecosystem while delivering quality health care.

—Elizabeth Plourde - 2003

Resource List

Support Groups, Information, and Bulletin Boards:

The Coalition for Post Tubal Women (CPT Women)
1629 S. Hamilton - Suite 200
Lockport, IL 60441
815 834-0987
www.tubal.org

HERS Foundation
(Hysterectomy Education Research Service)
Nora Coffey, Director
422 Bryn Mawr Avenue
Bala Cynwyd, PA 19004
610 667-7757
888 750-4377
www.hersfoundation.com
info@hersfoundation.com

Hyster Sister's Website for Hysterectomy Support
Hyster Sisters, Inc.
2436 S. I-35 E. Suite 376-184,
Denton, Texas 76205-4900
www.hystersisters.com
info@hystersisters.com

National Uterine Fibroid Foundation (NUFF)
Carla Dionne, Director
PO Box 9688
Colorado Springs, CO 80932-0688
719 633-3454
877 553-6833
www.nuff.org

Sans-Uteri Internet support group
Beth Tiner, Founder findings@findings.net
1621 Glyndon Avenue
Venice CA, 90291-2923
310 399-4849
www.findings.net
findings@findings.net

WebMD
www.webmd.com

Reading List

A Gynecologist's Second Opinion: The Questions and Answers You Need to Take Charge of Your Health, rev. ed., by William H. Parker, M.D. and Rachel L. Parker, et. al., Plume, 2003.

A Woman's Guide to Natural Hormones, by Christine Conrad, Perigee, 2000.

Anatomy of the Spirit: The Seven Stages of Power and Healing, by Caroline Myss, Ph.D., Random House, 1997.

Coping with Endometriosis: Sound, Compassionate Advice for Alleviating the Physical and Emotional Symptoms of This Frequently Misunderstood Disease, by Robert Phillips, Ph.D. and Glenda Motta, R.N., Avery, 2000.

Empowering Women: Every Woman's Guide to Successful Living, by Louise Hay, Hay House, 1999.

Estrogen, by Lila Nachtigall, M.D. and Joan Rattner Heilman, HarperPerennial, 1991.

Estrogen: How and Why It Can Save Your Life, by Adam Romoff, M.D., and Ina L. Yalof, Golden Books Pub., 1999.

Explaining Endometriosis, by Lorraine Henderson and Ros Wood, Allen & Unwin, 2000.

For Women Only: A Revolutionary Guide to Overcoming Sexual Dysfunction and Reclaiming Your Sex Life, Jennifer Berman, M.D., Laura Berman, Ph.D., and Elisabeth Bumiller, Henry Holt & Co. LLC, 2001.

For Women Only: Your Guide to Health Empowerment, Gary Null and Barbara Seaman, Seven Stories Press, 2001.

Health, Happiness & Hormones: One Woman's Journey Toward Health After a Hysterectomy, by Arlene Swaney, Starburst, 1996.

Heart Sense for Women: Your Plan for Natural Prevention and Treatment, by Stephen T. Sinatra, M.D., LifeLine Press, 2000.

Hormones and the Mind: A Woman's Guide to Enhancing Mood, Memory, and Sexual Vitality, by Edward L. Klaiber, M.D., HarperCollins Publishers, 2001.

It's My OVARIES, Stupid!, by Elizabeth Lee Vliet, M.D., Scribner, 2003.

Menopause & Mid-life Health, by Morris Notelovitz, M.D., Ph.D. and Diana Tonnessen, St. Martin's Press, 1994.

Misinformed Consent: Women's Stories about Unnecessary Hysterectomy, rev. ed., by Lise Cloutier-Steele, Next Decade, 2003.

Menopause & Mid-life Health, by Morris Notelovitz, M.D., Ph.D. and Diana Tonnessen, St. Martin's Press, 1994.

Natural Hormone Balance for Women: Look Younger, Feel Stronger, and Live Life with Exuberance, Uzzi Reiss, M.D. and Martin Zucker, Pocket Books, 2001.

Natural Hormone Replacement: For Women Over 45, by Jonathan Wright, M.D. and John Morgenthaler, Smart Publications, 1997.

No More Hysterectomies, by Vickie Hufnagel, M.D. with Susan Golant, NAL Penguin, 1988.

Our Health, Our Lives: A Revolutionary Approach to Total Health Care for Women, by Eileen Hoffman, M.D., Pocket Books, 1996.

Quantum Healing, by Deepak Chopra, M.D., Bantam Book, 1989.

Screaming to be Heard: Hormone Connections Women Suspect and Doctors Ignore, rev. ed., by Elizabeth Lee Vliet, M.D., M. Evans & Co., 2001.

Severed Trust: Why American Medicine Hasn't Been Fixed-and What We Can Do About It, by George D. Lundberg, M.D. and James H. Stacey, Basic Books, 2002.

Sex, Lies & the Truth about Uterine Fibroids: A Journey from Diagnosis to Treatment to Renewed Good Health, by Carla Dionne, Avery, 2001.

The Case Against Hysterectomy, by Sandra Simkin, Rivers Oram Press/Pandora List, 1998.

The Change Before the Change: Everything You Need to Know to Stay Healthy in the Decade Before Menopause, by Laura Corio, M.D. and Linda Kahn, Bantam Books, 2000.

The Creation of Health: The Emotional, Psychological, and Spiritual Responses That Promote Health and Healing, by Caroline Myss, Ph.D. and C. Norman Shealy, M.D., Ph.D., Three Rivers Press, 1998.

The Endometriosis Answer Book: New Hope, New Help, by Niels Lauersen, M.D., Ph.D. and Constance de Swaan, Fawcett Colombine Book, 1988.

The Estrogen Decision Self Help Book: The Most Up-to-date and Complete Guide for Relief of Menopausal Symptoms through Hormonal Replacement and Alternative Therapies, by Susan Lark, M.D., Celestial Arts, 1996.

The Hormone of Desire: The Truth about Testosterone, Sexuality, and Menopause, by Susan Rako, M.D., Three Rivers Press, 1996.

The Hysterectomy Hoax, by Stanley West, M.D., West, 2000.

The No-Hysterectomy Option: Your Body-Your Choice, by Herbert A. Goldfarb, M.D. with Judith Greif, John Wiley & Sons, 1990.

The Osteoporosis Solution: New Therapies for Prevention and Treatment, Carl Germano R.D., C.N.S., L.D.N., Kensington Books, 1999.

The Other Choice: A Comprehensive Guide for Women with Fibroids, by Sophie Bartsich, Ernst Bartsich, M.D., Xlibris Corporation, 2000.

The Pause: Positive Approaches to Perimenopause and Menopause, by Lonnie Barbach, Ph.D., Plume, 2000.

The V Book: A Doctor's Guide to Complete Vulvovaginal Health, by Elizabeth G. Stewart and Paul Spencer, Bantam Doubleday Dell Pub., 2002.

The Wisdom of Menopause: Creating Physical and Emotional Health and Healing during the Change, Christiane Northrup, M.D., Bantam Doubleday Dell Pub., 2001.

What Women Need to Know: From Headaches to Heart Disease and Everything in Between, by Marianne Legato, M.D. and Carol Colman, Olmstead Press, 2000.

What Your Doctor May Not Tell You about Menopause: The Breakthrough Book on Natural Progesterone, by John Lee, M.D. with Virginia Hopkins, Warner Books, 1996.

What Your Doctor May Not Tell You about Premenopause: Balance Your Hormones and Your Life from Thirty to Fifty, by John Lee, M.D., Jesse Hanley, M.D., Virginia Hopkins, Warner Books, 1999.

Women's Bodies, Women's Wisdom, by Christiane Northrup, M.D., Bantam Books, 1994.

Women, Weight and Hormones, by Elizabeth Lee Vliet, M.D., M. Evans & Co., 2001.

You Can Heal Your Life, by Louise Hay, Hay House, 1984.

You Don't Have to Live with Cystitis, by Larrian Gillespie, M.D., Avon Books, 1996.

You Don't Need a Hysterectomy: New and Effective Ways of Avoiding Major Surgery, by Ivan Strausz, M.D., Perseus Publishing, 2001.

Your Guide to Hysterectomy, Ovary Removal, & Hormone Replacement, by Elizabeth Plourde, C.L.S., M.A., New Voice Publications, 2002.

Glossary

17beta-estradiol/17b-estradiol/estradiol: the most potent, naturally occurring human estrogen. Manufactured primarily in the ovaries, it is predominantly found in the body before menopause.

Abdominal hysterectomy: removal of the uterus through a cut in the abdominal wall.

Adenomyosis: benign growth of glands inside the uterus growing into the muscular wall of the uterus.

Alzheimer's disease: a form of brain disease. It can lead to confusion, memory loss, restlessness, problems with perception, speech trouble, trouble moving, and fearing things that are not there. Breakdown of the cells of the brain does occur.

Androgens: any steroid hormone that promotes the development and maintenance of male or masculine characteristics, present in both men and women. Also see testosterone.

Androstenedione: steroid produced by the ovary, testis, and adrenal cortex which can be converted into testosterone and/or estrogens.

Anti-depressant: any drug used to alleviate depression by altering chemicals in the brain.

Bi-est: estriol and estradiol combined in creams or sublinguals.

Bilateral oophorectomy: removal of both ovaries.

Bowel prolapse: see prolapsed bowel.

BSO (bilateral salpingo-oophorectomy): removal of both fallopian tubes and ovaries.

Carcinoma-in-situ: precancerous condition usually of the cervix.

Castration: the removal of one or both ovaries or testicles.

Cellular irregularities: abnormal changes in size, shape, and organization within cells.

Cervix: the lower portion, or neck of the uterus.

CIN I, II, III: ranking of severity of cellular abnormalities of the cervix. I is considered mild and III is severe.

Clinical Laboratory Scientist (C.L.S.): a person, who upon completing a Bachelor's degree in the biological sciences, a one year hospital internship, and passes state testing then qualifies to be licensed by the state (in California) to perform and report laboratory analysis on blood and body fluids.

Colonoscopy/coloscopy: visual examination of the colon using a colonoscope (an endoscope which is usually a fiber-optic tube).

Corpus luteum cysts: hormone body formed at site of ruptured mature egg follicle, which secretes estrogen and progesterone. It normally regresses and is shed at menstruation.

Cryotherapy: therapeutic use of cold to destroy abnormal tissue.

CT Scans (computerized tomography): a technique utilized for examining internal structures of the body.

Cystocele: herniation of the bladder into the front wall of the vagina.

Cystourethrapexy: surgical repair of the bladder and urethra.

D&C/dilation and curettage: a procedure whereby the cervix is dilated or stretched to allow curettement, or scraping of the endometrium, or lining of the uterus.

Deprivation: a lack of something that is essential for physical or mental well-being.

DHEA: dehydroepiandrosterone; an adrenal hormone with weak androgen effects that is a precursor to testosterone. It is the major androgen precursor in females and postmenopausal women.

Diabetes: a disease affecting sugar use by the body; characterized by excessive urination and thirst.

Diverticulosis/diverticulitis: inflammation of pouches in the wall of the colon.

Dysfunction: disturbance, impairment, or abnormality of the functioning of a body organ or system.

Dysmenorrhea: painful menstrual periods.

Dysplasia: abnormal tissue development due to changes in size, shape, and organization within cells.

Endocrine (organ) gland: a ductless gland that releases hormones directly into the blood. They affect the function of specific target organs and exert powerful influences on growth, sexual development, and metabolism.

Endometrial ablation: surgical cauterization of the lining of the uterus.
Endometrial cancer: cancer of the lining of the uterus.

Endometriosis: the abnormal occurrence of tissue which resembles the endometrium (lining of the uterus) in various locations in the pelvic cavity, including the uterine wall, ovaries, or extragenital sites.

ERT: estrogen replacement therapy.

Estradiol: see 17beta-estradiol.

Estriol: a relatively weak, naturally occurring human estrogen. Primarily produced by the placenta during pregnancy, throughout the rest of women's lives, it is a metabolite of 17beta-estradiol and estrone.

Estrogen (oestrogen): name given to a group of hormones produced by the ovaries, testis, placenta, and possibly the adrenal cortex; responsible for female sexual characteristics. The three important human forms, ranked in order of potency, are estradiol, estrone, and estriol.

Estrone: one of the body's natural estrogens, which is less potent than 17beta-estradiol. It is manufactured primarily in the fat, muscle, and skin tissues by conversion of the ovary's estradiol, or the male hormones, androstenedione and testosterone. It is the predominant form of estrogen found in the body after menopause.

Fibroids/Fibroid tumors: (fibroid tumors/leiomyomata/myomata) benign tumors which stem from the smooth muscle of the uterus. A common cause for heavy bleeding in women.

Fibromyalgia: a syndrome whose symptoms include widespread muscle pain, persistent fatigue, generalized morning stiffness, multiple tender points, and non-refreshing sleep.

Gynecologist: physician specializing in the care and treatment of women and their diseases, especially those affecting the sexual organs.

HMO: Health Maintenance Organization; these provide managed health care for groups.

Hormone: a chemical messenger produced in organs of the body, transported by the blood, and having a specific regulatory effect on the activity of certain cells or organs remote from its origin.

Hot flushes/hot flashes: also called hot flashes, temporary rises in body temperature, primarily associated with menopause.

HRT: hormone replacement therapy.

Hypertension: the medical term for high blood pressure.

Hysterectomy: total or partial surgical removal of the uterus.

Hysteroscopy: inspection of the inside lining of the uterus with an endoscope inserted through the cervix from the vagina.

IC: see interstitial cystitis.

Ilioinguinal: pertaining to the iliac (or a portion of the small intestine) and groin region.

Incontinence: the inability or failure to hold or control one's urine or feces.

Insulin: protein hormone made by the islets of Langerhans in the pancreas. It participates, together with other chemicals, in regulating carbohydrate and fat metabolism. It checks the accumulation of glucose in the blood and promotes the utilization of sugar in the treatment of diabetes.

Interstitial cystitis (IC): a bladder inflammation, characterized by an inflamed, ulcerated, and scarred bladder wall, which occurs almost exclusively in women; producing symptoms similar to urinary infection, including urinary urgency, day and night frequency, and pain.

Irritable bowel syndrome (IBS): abnormally increased motility (spontaneous movement) of small and large intestines, accompanied by pain and diarrhea.

Laparoscope: a long slender instrument used for the visual examination of the interior of a body cavity.

Laparoscopic hysterectomy: a procedure for removing the uterus with the aid of a laparoscope.

LEEP/Loop electrocautery excision procedure: an electrically charged wire loop used to cauterize abnormal tissue.

Leiomyoma/leiomyoma/leiomyomata: a benign tumor derived from smooth muscle, most commonly the uterus, also called fibroids.

Lipids: any one of a group of fats or fat-like substances. Technically, it is a general term for a number of different water-insoluble compounds found in the body.

LSO (left salpingo-oophorectomy): left fallopian tube and ovary removal.

Lyse/lysis: destruction of cells or tissue.

Menopause: physical loss of menstruation (periods), either as a normal part of aging, around the average age of 51.5, or as a result of surgery.

Menorrhagia: heavy menstrual flow.

Menstrual cycle: a woman's monthly reproductive cycle.

Menstruation: that part of a woman's menstrual cycle when the superficial two-thirds of the endometrium is shed as part of the menstrual flow.

Mittelschmerz: intermenstrual pain associated with ovulation.

Mortality: a fatal outcome, or death.

Myoma/myomas/myomata: a benign tumor made of muscular fiber in the uterus. Also see fibroids.

Myomectomy: surgical removal of a myoma or myomata, or uterine fibroids, while preserving the uterus.

Myometrial nodule: round mass in muscular wall of uterus.

Non-insulin-dependent diabetes mellitus (NIDDM): type II diabetes mellitus. An often mild form of diabetes of gradual onset with minimal and no symptoms of metabolic disturbance, with no requirement for insulin. Peak age of onset is 50 to 60 years. Obesity and possibly a genetic factor are usually present.

Ob-gyn/obstetrician-gynecologist: a physician specializing in pregnancy, childbirth, and female reproductive physiology.

Oestrogen: see estrogen.

Oophorectomy/ovariectomy: surgery to remove one or both of the ovaries. Also known as ovariectomy or castration.

Oophorohysterectomy: the surgical removal of the ovaries and uterus.

Osteoporosis: a decrease in bone tissue with a reduction in bone mass along with increased interior space (small holes), resulting in thinning, demineralization, and weakening of the bones, making them more vulnerable to breakage from minimal trauma; sometimes accompanied by pain and/or body deformity.

Ovarian cyst: a small sack filled with fluid or semisolid material that grows in or on the ovary.

Ovariectomy: see oophorectomy.

Ovaries: the female gonads or reproductive glands, that correspond to the male testicles. Their function is to store and release eggs and to manufacture hormones.

Pap smear: test used as a screening for cervical cancer and can also detect vaginal cancer.

Partial hysterectomy: see subtotal hysterectomy.

Pelvic inflammatory disease: inflammation or infection within the pelvic cavity.

Perimenopausal/Premenopausal: the three to five years before the menopause and when estrogen levels start dropping.

PID: see pelvic inflammatory disease.

Plaque: a patch of fatty build-up on the lining of a blood vessel. Atherosclerosis of the arteries.

PMS: see premenstrual syndrome.

Polyp: a protruding growth that comes out from the mucous membrane.

Postmenopausal: occurring after the menopause.

Postoperative/post-op: time following an operation.

Premarin®: a brand name for conjugated equine estrogens collected from pregnant mares' urine.

Premenopausal: see perimenopausal.

Premenstrual syndrome (PMS): the diagnostic term used to describe a variety of physical, psychological, and emotional symptoms occurring just prior to menstrual flow (periods).

Progesterone: a steroid hormone produced by the ovary after ovulation takes place which prepares the uterus for implantation of a fertilized ovum (egg). It is essential for pregnancy, during which time it reaches levels 300 times normal. It is utilized in HRT and in the management of various ovarian disorders; excessive bleeding, amenorrhea (lack of periods), etc.

Progestin: see progestogen/progestagen/progestin.

Progestogen/Progestagen/Progestin: a term applied to any substance possessing progesterone-like activity: either natural progesterone, or a modified form having similar actions (synthetic progesterone), which produces changes in the uteral endometrium (lining of uterus). Synthetic forms produce biological responses which are different than natural progesterone. One primary utilization is in birth control pills.

Prolapsed bowel: see rectocele.

Prolapsed uterus: the falling down of the uterus in varying degrees: from the cervix falling within the vaginal cavity, to the entire uterus outside the vagina.

Prophylactic: a procedure that prevents or helps to prevent the development of disease.

Prophylactic ovarian removal: the surgical removal of the ovaries utilized as a preventive measure against possible cancer.

Prozac®: a brand name for fluoxetine, an antidepressant which works by increasing available serotonin levels.

Rectocele: herniation of the rectum into the back wall of the vagina; prolapse of the bowel.

Reproductive organs: the male and female sex glands. In women these include the ovaries, fallopian tubes, and uterus.

RSO (right salpingo-oophorectomy): right fallopian tube and ovary removal.

Serotonin (5-HT): a brain neurotransmitter produced from tryptophan, which is found in high quantities in many body tissues, including the intestinal mucosa, pineal body, and central nervous system. It has multiple biologic effects in the body, including regulation of sleep, body temperature, blood pressure, learning, appetite, intestinal motility, pain perception, sexual behavior, reduces the breakdown of collagen, inhibits gastrointestinal secretion, and stimulates smooth muscle. Increasing its level is the basis of antidepressant therapy. Also called 5-HT, or 5-hydroxytryptamine.

Sublingual: beneath the tongue.

Subtotal hysterectomy: the surgical removal of the body of the uterus, leaving the cervix in place.

Supracervical hysterectomy: see subtotal hysterectomy.

Supravaginal hysterectomy: see subtotal hysterectomy.

Surgical menopause: ending of menstruation due to the surgical removal of the uterus. More commonly used to denote the menopausal state brought on by surgical removal of the ovaries and/or uterus.

TAH: total abdominal hysterectomy.

Testosterone: the major androgenic hormone associated with male secondary sexual characteristics; produced by the testicles and ovaries.

Thyroid: endocrine gland located at the neck just below the larynx, extending around the front and to either side of the trachea (windpipe). It secretes the hormones thyroxine (T4), and triiodothyronine (T3), both vital to growth and metabolism.

Thyroid hormones: hormones produced and released by the thyroid gland. Also see thyroid.

Total hysterectomy: the surgical removal of both the cervix and the body of the uterus.

Tri-est: estriol, estradiol and estrone.

Tubal ligation: also called tubal sterilization. Involves the blocking of the fallopian tubes as a means of birth-control. There are different methods: early methods involved cutting, tying, and burning of the tubes; more recent methods include microsurgery, and clipping the tubes.

TVH: total vaginal hysterectomy.

UAE (uterine artery embolization): a procedure performed to shrink fibroid tumors which utilizes small plastic particles to block the blood flow to the uterus and tumor.

Unilateral-salpingo-oophorectomy (USO): removal of one fallopian tube and ovary.

Ureter: one of a pair of tubes that carry urine from the kidneys into the bladder.

Ureteral: of, or pertaining to the ureter.

Urethra: small tubular structure that drains urine from the bladder.

Urethral: of, or pertaining to the urethra.

Urinary incontinence: difficulty in retaining urine. Also see incontinence.

Urogynecologist: a physician specializing in diagnosis and treatment of diseases of the genitourinary tract and reproductive organs.

USO: see unilateral-salpingo-oophorectomy.

Uterine prolapse: see prolapsed uterus.

Uterus: the womb of a woman. A pear-shaped hollow, thick-walled muscular organ that houses the developing fetus. It is becoming recognized as an endocrine (hormone) producing organ.

Vagina/Vaginal: a muscular tube about three inches long connecting the uterine cervix with the external female genitals.

Vaginal hysterectomy: removal of the uterus through the vagina, without cutting the wall of the abdomen.

Vaginal prolapse: the falling of the vagina, which can lead to its outward protrusion.

Notes

1   43% of hysterectomized women experience considerable deterioration in their bowel habits. van Dam JH, Gosselink MJ, et al. "Changes in bowel function after hysterectomy." *Dis Colon Rectum*. 1997. 40:1342-7.

"Constipation, interrupted defecation, and defecation disorders in general are unfortunately common findings after hysterectomy." Wiersma TjG, Werre AJ, et al. "Hysterectomy: the anorectal pitfall." *Scand Jour Gastroenterol*. 1997. 32(suppl)223:3-7. See also Elizabeth Plourde. *Your Guide to Hysterectomy, Ovary Removal, & Hormone Replacement*. Chapter 11 - "Bladder and Bowel Problems: Increased Risk." New Voice Publications 2002. pp142-149.

2   Loss of the uterus, and its contractions during orgasm, alters the sensations and reactions that some women are used to experiencing during sex. Masters WH, Johnson VE. "The female orgasm." In: *Human sexual response*. Boston, MA. Little Brown & Co. 1966. Ch. 9 pp127-140. Masters WH, Johnson VE. "Similarities in physiologic response." In: *Human sexual response*. Boston, MA. Little Brown & Co. 1966. Ch. 13 p. 288. Fox CA, Wolff HS, Baker JA. "Measurement of intra-vaginal and intra-uterine pressures during human coitus by radiotelemetry." *Jour Reprod Fert*. 1970. 22:243-251.

When women undergo both a hysterectomy and oophorectomy, they report a waning of libido (sexual desire), when compared with hysterectomized patients whose ovaries are preserved. Nathorst-

Boos J, von Schoultz B, Carlstrom K. "Elective ovarian removal and estrogen replacement therapy—effects on sexual life, psychological well-being and androgen status." *Jour Psy Obstet Gynecol*. 1993 Dec. 14(4):283-93.

Oophorectomized women complain of a deteriorated sex life, expressing that they experience less pleasure from sex, an impaired sex drive, and decreased lubrication. Nathorst-Boos J, von Schoultz B, Carlstrom K. "Elective ovarian removal and estrogen replacement therapy—effects on sexual life, psychological well-being and androgen status." *Jour Psy Obstet Gynecol*. 1993 Dec. 14(4):283-93. Bellerose SB; Binik YM. "Body image and sexuality in oophorectomized women." *Archives of Sexual Behavior*. 1993 Oct. 22(5):435-459. Nathorst-Boos J, von Schoultz B. "Psychological reactions and sexual life after hysterectomy with and without oophorectomy." *Gynecol Obstet Invest*. 1992. 34:97-101.

Conflicting results show that when women opt for removal of their reproductive organs they gamble with the quality of their lives. Even though 8 to 12% of women state their sex life improved after surgery, a number of studies show that an average of 30% of hysterectomized and/or oophorectomized women are not able to enjoy sex the same as before the operation. Kretzschmar NR, Gardiner S. "A consideration of the surgical menopause after hysterectomy and the occurrence of cancer in the stump following subtotal hysterectomy." *Amer Jour Obstet Gynecol*. 1935. 29:168-175. Filiberti A, Regazzoni M, Garavoglia M, Perilli C, Alpinelli P, et al. "Problems after hysterectomy. A comparative content analysis of 60 interviews with cancer and non-cancer hysterectomized women." *Eur Jour Gynaec Oncol*. 1991. XII(6):445-9. Kilkku P, Gronroos M, Hirvonen T, Rauramo L. "Supravaginal uterine amputation vs. hysterectomy: effects on libido and orgasm." *Acta Obstet Gynecol Scand*. 1983. 62:147-152. Nathorst-Boos J, von Schoultz B. "Psychological reactions and sexual life after hysterectomy with and without oophorectomy." *Gynecol Obstet Invest.* 1992. 34:97-101. Raboch J, Boudnik V, Raboch J Jr. "Sex life following hysterectomy." *Geburtshilfe Frauenheilkd.* 1985 Jan. 45(1):48-50. (Abstract). See also Elizabeth Plourde. *Your Guide to Hysterectomy, Ovary Removal, & Hormone Replacement.* Chapter 13 - "Sexual Enjoyment: Where did it go?" New Voice Publications 2002. pp158-168.

3   Hysterectomized women have a 40% higher prevalence of daily urinary incontinence, when compared to women who have not had a hysterectomy. Researchers finding that hysterectomies, along with obesity, are the highest preventable risk factors associated with incontinence conclude: "Our finding that hysterectomy may independently increase the prevalence of urinary incontinence 20-30 years later should encourage reevaluation of the indications for hysterectomy and further study of alternative treatments for benign conditions." Brown JS, Seeley DG, et al. "Urinary incontinence in older women: who is at risk?" *Obstet Gynecol.* 1996 May. 87(5)(part 1):715-721. See also Elizabeth Plourde. *Your Guide to Hysterectomy, Ovary Removal, & Hormone Replacement.* Chapter 11 - "Bladder and Bowel Problems: Increased Risk." New Voice Publications 2002. pp142-149.

4   The death rate for this surgery when performed for non life-threatening conditions, is between 0.06 and 0.2% (or 6 to 20 deaths in every 10,000 operations). Boyd ME, Groome PA. "The morbidity of abdominal hysterectomy." *Canadian Jour Surg.* 1993 Apr. 36(2):155-9. Chryssikopoulos A, Loghis C. "Indications and results of total hysterectomy." *Int Surg.* 1986. 71:188-194. Wingo PA, Huezo CM, Rubin GL, et al. "The mortality risk associated with hysterectomy." *Amer Jour Obstet Gynecol.* 1985 Aug 1. 152(7 pt 1): 803-8.

With 22 million performed in America since 1965, the death rate translates into between 12,000 to 40,000 women who have died just as a result of their surgery. Pokras R, Hufnagel VG. "Hysterectomies in the United States, 1965-84: Data from the National Health Survey." In: *Vital & Health Statistics*. Washington, D.C.: U.S. CDC. Series 13, number 92. pp1-31. Lepine LA, Hillis SD, Marchbanks PA, et al. "Hysterectomy surveillance—United States, 1980-1993." *MMWR*, U.S. Centers For Disease Control. 1997 Aug. 46(SS-4):1-15. "National Center for Health Statistics: Utilization of short-stay hospitals: Annual summary for the United States." [Current title: National Hospital Discharge Survey: Annual Summary.] In: *Vital & Health Statistics*. Washington, D.C. [Multiple years 1973-2000]. Series 13, numbers 24,26,31,37,41,60,61,64,72,78,83,84,91,96,99, 106,109,112,119,121,128,133,140,144,148,151,&153. Popovic JR, Kozak LJ. "National hospital discharge survey: Annual summary, 1998." In: *Vital & Health Statistics*. Hyattsville, MD: National Center for Health Statistics. 2000 Sept. 13(148). Table 27. p33. [Note: 1965-2000 Actual and 2001-2002 projected estimate.]

5   In the United States, 12.2% of hysterectomies, or approximately 79,000 women undergo hysterectomy for chronic pelvic pain every year. Dicker RC, Greenspan JR, Strauss LT, Cowart MR, et al. "Complications of abdominal and vaginal hysterectomy among women of reproductive age in the United States: The Collaborative Review of Sterilization." *Amer Jour Obstet Gynecol*. 1982 Dec. 144(7):841-8. Popovic JR, Kozak LJ. "National hospital discharge survey: Annual summary, 1998." In: *Vital & Health Statistics*. Hyattsville, MD: National Center for Health Statistics. 2000 Sept. 13(148). Table 27. p33.

For 22%, or approximately 17,000, surgery does not provide relief from their chronic pelvic pain. Stovall TG, Ling FW, et al. "Hysterectomy for chronic pelvic pain of presumed uterine etiology." *Obstet Gynecol*. 1990. 75:676-9. Smith RP. "Pelvic Pain." In: *Gynecology in Primary Care*. Baltimore, MD. Williams & Wilkins. 1997. Ch. 22 p494.

6   When specifically looking at whether estrogen influences memory, studies on both ovariectomized research animals and postmenopausal women confirm that estrogen therapy does increase memory and protect against memory decline. Simpkins JW, Green PS, Gridley KE, et al. "Role of estrogen replacement therapy in memory enhancement and the prevention of neuronal loss associated with Alzheimer's disease." *Amer Jour Med.* 1997 Sept. 103(3A):19S-25S. Resnick SM, Metter EJ, Zonderman AB. "Estrogen replacement therapy and longitudinal decline in visual memory: a possible protective effect?" *Neurology.* 1997 Dec. 49:1491-7. Henderson VW, Watt L, Buckwalter JG. "Cognitive skills associated with estrogen replacement in women with Alzheimer's disease." *Psychoneuroendocrinology.* 1996. 21(4):421-430.

When testing postmenopausal women who receive both estrogen and progestin, they commit 40% fewer errors on both verbal and spatial working memory tasks compared to non-users. Duff SJ, Hampson E. "A beneficial effect of estrogen on working memory in postmenopausal women taking hormone replacement therapy." *Hormones and Behavior.* 2000 Dec. 38(4):262-276. See also Elizabeth Plourde. *Your Guide to Hysterectomy, Ovary Removal, & Hormone Replacement.* Chapter 15 - "Social, Political & Economic Institutions" New Voice Publications 2002. pp192-195.

7   When only one ovary is left, there is a great possibility that it will shut down. This result is so common, one research article concluded with: "The fact that one-third of the patients undergoing USO (one ovary removed) will develop ovarian dysfunction raises the question whether there is a place for this procedure." Bukovsky I, Halperin R, Schneider D, Golan A, Hertzianu I, Herman A. "Ovarian function following abdominal hysterectomy with and without unilateral oophorectomy." *Eur Jour Obstet Gynecol Repro Biol.* 1995 Jan. 58(1):29-32. See also Elizabeth Plourde. *Your Guide to Hysterectomy, Ovary Removal, & Hormone Replacement.* Chapter 3 -

"The Ovaries: Finely tuned, essential chemical manufacturing plants." New Voice Publications 2002. pp46-59.

8   The hormones of the hypothalamus-pituitary-adrenal (HPA) axis interact with the gonadal (sex) hormones causing spurts of hormones to release throughout the day and night. This is a crucial factor for the normal functioning of the body in everyday life. Disrupted pulse patterns are connected to many disorders, including jet lag, inability to sleep, and depression. Van Cauter E, Turek FW. "Endocrine and other biological rhythms." In: *Endocrinology*, eds. DeGroot LJ, et al. 3rd ed. Philadelphia, PA. WB Saunders Co. 1995. Vol 3 Ch. 140 pp2487-2548.

Low levels of estradiol are linked to poor sleep; while the secretion of GH is tightly associated with the beginning of the sleep period in normal adults. Hollander LE, Freeman EW, Sammel MD, et al. "Sleep quality, estradiol levels, and behavioral factors in late reproductive age women." *Obstet Gynecol.* 2001 Sept. 98(3):391-7. Van Cauter E, Turek FW. "Endocrine and other biological rhythms." In: *Endocrinology*, eds. DeGroot LJ, et al. 3rd ed. Philadelphia, PA. WB Saunders Co. 1995. Vol 3 Ch. 140 p2502. See also Elizabeth Plourde. *Your Guide to Hysterectomy, Ovary Removal, & Hormone Replacement.* Chapter 9 - "Depression: I can't get out of the house." New Voice Publications 2002. pp122-136.

9   Estrogen's antidepressive actions prove that the depression women experience after their hysterectomy has a biochemical basis. Ditkoff EC, Crary WG, Cristo M, Lobo RA. "Estrogen improves psychological function in asymptomatic postmenopausal women." *Obstet Gynecol.* 1991 Dec. 78(6):991-5. Sherwin BB, Gelfand MM. "Sex steroids and affect in the surgical menopause: a double-blind, cross-over study." *Psychoneuroendocrinology.* 1985. 10(3):325-335. Barker MG. "Psychiatric illness after hysterectomy." *Brit Med Jour.* 1968 April 13. 2:91-5. A Dictionary of Psychological Medicine.

1892. Vol II. s.v. "Ovariotomy and oophorectomy in relation to insanity and epilepsy." Bantock GG. "Hysterectomy and insanity." *Brit Med Jour.* 1889 Aug 17. 2:395-6. Ananth J. "Hysterectomy and depression." *Obstet Gynecol.* 1978 Dec. 52(6):724-730. See also Elizabeth Plourde. *Your Guide to Hysterectomy, Ovary Removal, & Hormone Replacement.* Chapter 9 - "Depression: I can't get out of the house." New Voice Publications 2002. pp122-136.

10   When tested for extroversion (the ability to be socially self-confident and involved in the affairs of others), women given estrogen exhibited significant gains in their scores, whereas the scores of those receiving placebos showed a decrease. (These results demonstrate that estrogen deficiency does have an effect on women's ability to be around people and emotionally connect with them.) Fedor-Freybergh P. "The influence of oestrogens on the well being and mental performance in climacteric and postmenopausal women." *Acta Obstet Gyn Scand.* 1977. 64(S):1-68.

11   Articles connecting hysterectomies to atherosclerosis have been published in medical journals since the 1950s. In 1981, one doctor concluded: "Pending further elucidation of the relationship between hysterectomy and cardiovascular disease, gynecologists should consider advising premenopausal women who are considering hysterectomy on the risks of coronary heart disease following the procedure." Centerwall BS. "Premenopausal hysterectomy and cardiovascular disease." *Amer Jour Obstet Gynecol.* 1981 Jan 1. 139(1):58-61.

"In any case, physicians in practice should recognize the potential of the uterus as a systemically active organ whose removal significantly increases subsequent risk of myocardial infarction (heart attack)." Shelton JD. "Prostacyclin from the uterus and woman's cardiovascular advantage." *Prostaglandins Leukotrienes Med.* 1982. 8:459-466. See also Elizabeth Plourde. *Your Guide to*

Hysterectomy, Ovary Removal, & Hormone Replacement. Chapter 6 - "Atherosclerosis: Inevitable artery plaque build-up" New Voice Publications 2002. pp83-96.

12   36% of hysterectomized women exhibit high blood pressure, compared to 21% in the population as a whole. When hysterectomy is combined with oophorectomy, the percentage becomes 44%— more than double the general population. "The main finding of our study was that hysterectomy with ovarian preservation is associated with increased diastolic (minimum) blood pressure and the diagnosis of hypertension (high blood pressure)." Luoto R, Kaprio J, Reunanen A, Rutanen E-M. "Cardiovascular morbidity in relation to ovarian function after hysterectomy." *Obstet Gynecol.* 1995 Apr. 85(4):515-522. See also Elizabeth Plourde. *Your Guide to Hysterectomy, Ovary Removal, & Hormone Replacement.* Chapter 5 - "High Blood Pressure: Unknown risk" New Voice Publications 2002. pp71-82.

13   Between 14 to 28% of hysterectomized women report having a problem with either weight gain or loss after surgery. Gould D. "Hidden problems after a hysterectomy." *Nursing Times.* 1986 June. 82(23):43-6. Luoto R, Kaprio J, Reunanen A, Rutanen E-M. "Cardiovascular morbidity in relation to ovarian function after hysterectomy." *Obstet Gynecol.* 1995 Apr. 85(4):515-522. Hysterectomy, even with ovarian preservation, is associated with weight gain. Luoto R, Kaprio J, Reunanen A, Rutanen E-M. "Cardiovascular morbidity in relation to ovarian function after hysterectomy." *Obstet Gynecol.* 1995 Apr. 85(4):515-522.